IOI
POWER
CRYSTALS

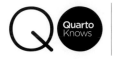

Quarto is the authority on a wide range of topics.

Quarto educates, entertains and enriches the lives of our readers—enthusiasts and lovers of hands-on living.

www.QuartoKnows.com

© 2011 Fair Winds Press
Text © 2011 Judy Hall

First published in the USA in 2011 by
Fair Winds Press, an imprint of
Quarto Publishing Group USA Inc.
100 Cummings Center
Suite 406-L
Beverly, MA 01915-6101
Telephone: (978) 282-9590
Fax: (978) 283-2742
QuartoKnows.com
Visit our blogs at QuartoKnows.com

17   13

ISBN-13: 978-1-59233-490-2

Digital edition published in 2011
eISBN: 978-1-61058-151-6

Library of Congress Cataloging-in-Publication Data is available

Cover image: Trigonic Quartz
Cover design by Kathie Alexander
Book design by Kathie Alexander
Photography by Exquisite Crystals, www.exquisitecrystals.com, except for: page 9: Carsten Peter/Speleoresearch & Films/National Geographic/Getty Images; page 13: © ian woolcock / Alamy; page 14: © Geo Images / Alamy

Printed and bound in China

No medical claims are made for the stones in this book and the information given is not intended to act as a substitute for medical treatment. If you have any doubt about their use, consult a qualified crystal-healing practitioner. In the context of this book, illness is a dis-ease, the final manifestation of spiritual, environmental, psychological, karmic, emotional or mental imbalance, blockage, or distress. Healing means bringing mind, body, and spirit back into balance and facilitating evolution for the soul; it does not imply a cure. In accordance with crystal-healing consensus, all stones are referred to as crystals, regardless of whether or not they have a crystalline structure.

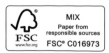

MIX
Paper from
responsible sources
FSC® C016973

101 POWER CRYSTALS

THE ULTIMATE GUIDE
TO MAGICAL CRYSTALS, GEMS, AND STONES
FOR HEALING AND TRANSFORMATION

JUDY HALL

The Power of Crystals

The wondrous lore that I prepare to show. For all the pests that out of the earth arise, the earth's ownself the antidote supplies. She breeds the viper, but she to the sage the means presents to quell the viper's rage. All kinds of gems spring from her bosom wide. And hapless mortals with sure help provide. For all what virtues potent herbs possession, gems in their kind have, nor in measure less. Great is the force . . . that in stones inherent are. For in the stone implanted mother earth external force, unfading, at its birth.
—*The Lithica*

Crystals have always been regarded as a source of power—and as a gift from the gods. Impressive no matter what their size, gems hold an aura of mystery and authority. From prehistory to the present, gemstones have symbolized wealth and been accorded wondrous properties. The ancient texts that tell us so much about the power of stones had their origins in the Stone Age, a time when technology quite literally came from stones. Since that time, we have continued to harness their magical power.

In 1714, M. B. Valentini's *Museum Museorum* pictured an airship designed five years earlier by a Brazilian priest; the craft was to be powered by Agate and iron that, when heated in the sun, would become magnetic. Strange as this may seem, our present-day technology could not exist without crystals; they power computers and surgical tools, coat automobile engines and spaceships. Crystals provide the basic building blocks of science and art.

The ancients credited crystals with healing power. The Greek philosopher Theophrastus and Roman geographer Pliny passed these remedies on (even though Pliny denounced some as false claims). The Babylonians attributed humankind's destiny to the influence of precious stones. Our ancestors believed the Earth was surrounded by crystal spheres where gods, stars, and planets dwelt. Originally a crystal's color or constitution or its planetary affiliation indicated its efficacy for specific conditions. Unfortunately, translation difficulties often make it impossible to ascertain exactly which stone early texts referred to, but some references are crystal clear.

Templates of Light

Each crystal has its own unique energy signature. These "templates of light" are encoded with all you need to activate your own power. The key is to find a crystal that is attuned to your own personal energy or that raises your energetic resonance to ensure well-being and expand your consciousness.

THE POWER OF GEMS

Not only flashy gemstones hold power. Since antiquity, crystals of all sorts have served as protective amulets. Humble stones such as Flint were magical carriers for the soul, for metaphysical workings, or for shamans to use on their otherworldly journeys. Many stones produced incandescent sparks or could be super-heated into streams of gold, silver, copper, and other precious metals. Just as magical were the sky rocks that fell to Earth, bringing with them iron to forge tools and create weapons.

Egyptologist Wallis Budge explained, "each stone possessed a sort of living personality, which could experience sickness and disease, and could become old and powerless and even die." However, in Egyptian medicine, stones could also heal. The Greek philosopher Plato believed stones were living beings, produced by a fermentation process induced by "a life-giving intelligence descending from the stars." According to many myths, crystals solidified from ice, a view reinforced by the bubbles of water sometimes found within a crystal.

The fifth-century Roman poet Claudian tells us that:

When the Alpine ice, frost-harden'd into stone
First braved the sun, and as a jewel shone,
Not all its substance could the gem assume—
Some tell-tale drops still linger'd in its womb.

HOW CRYSTALS FORM

Crystals are, for the most part, created by the Earth's awesome power. Boiled, compressed, and excoriated, some were born of volcanoes, glaciers, earthquakes, and immense pressure; others dripped into being through osmosis, gas bubbles, and nature's gentler forces.

Some so-called crystals don't actually have a crystalline structure. Amber, for instance, is fossilized tree resin, and volcanic Obsidian formed so fast it didn't have time to crystallize. How a crystal forms affects how its power works. Those that grew slowly tend to emit their power gently; those that were on an accelerated path of growth blast their power out to the world. Paradoxically, some of the youngest geological stones have the highest vibrations and the greatest power to transform our world.

The Power of Color

The power of color was first noted by the ancients and became an integral part of the magical healing processes by which imbalances were rectified and harmony restored. In 1878, Edwin D. Babbitt suggested color had therapeutic properties that could be applied in healing. His rationale may help to explain the power behind sympathetic magic and why particular colors traditionally were used to treat specific dis-eases. In Babbitt's "ray" system, red attracts iron, zinc, and Strontium; yellow sodium, phosphorous, and carbon; and so on. These minerals are required for correct functioning of the body. His chromatherapy was complex, and exposure to the colored rays needed to be carefully calibrated.

Crystal workers, though, simply utilize crystals of the appropriate color based on the ancient correspondences.

- Pink and peach stones heal emotional imbalances and gently energize your system.
- Red gems energize more forcefully and resonate with the reproductive system. Red also aids blood-related and inflammatory conditions.
- Orange is a mental and creative energizer, stimulating personal power and resonating with the Leydig gland above the testes, a seat of kundalini power.
- Yellow and gold stones are mental and nervous system stimulators; they resonate with neurotransmitters, the adrenal glands, and intestines, and balance your mind and emotions.
- Green is calming and associated with the heart, eyes, and thymus gland.
- Blue-green resonates with the subtle levels of being and opens metaphysical abilities.
- Blue resonates with the throat and thyroid gland, and has a tonic effect.
- Indigo has mystical qualities; it resonates with the pineal gland, but also effects mental healing.
- Violet and purple stones resonate with the pituitary, regulating metabolism and regenerating the body. They also open you to higher awareness.
- Black and brown stones detoxify and ground energy, protecting the body from harm.
- Combination stones synergize the effects of the colors and constituents.

The Power of Magic

For thrice seven days the mighty wizard fled the bath's refreshment and his consort's bed.
For thrice seven days a solemn fast maintained. Then in the living fount the gem he laves.
And in soft garments like an infant swathes. As to a god, he sacrifices brings.
And potent spells in mystic murmurs sings. Till moved by fervent prayer and mighty
charms, a living soul the prescient substance warms. Then in his hands he bears the thing di-
vine, where kindled lamps in his pure mansion shine. And as her infant son a mother holds,
so in his arms the talisman he folds. And thou, if thou wouldst hear the mystic voice, thus do,
and in the wondrous thing rejoice.—The Lithica

Crystals have always been credited with possessing magical power, as the above
quotation from a third-century B.C.E. stone book shows. It also describes the
awe and reverence with which they were handled. Magic isn't mere superstition—
it is the foundation for the experimental sciences that the modern world values
so highly. Without magic we would not have medicine, astronomy, literature and
drama, chemistry, mathematics, music, mythology, and perhaps even religion itself.
Magical formulae constitute some of the oldest writings, and it could be argued
that the alphabet—even the recording of knowledge itself—is a form of magic.
Magic isn't just a set of practices and beliefs; it is a way of looking at the world. The
view that the natural world was animate, alive with magical forces interpenetrating
the substance of the physical and the metaphysical realms, governed ancient life
and death. Crystal workers today still interact with the animate forces, the living
beings, within crystals.

The word *magic* comes from *magi*, the wise men and women of Persia and Baby-
lon, but has its roots in the Sumerian word *imga* meaning "deep" or "profound."
Magic was a way of manipulating the everyday world and attracting the favor of the
gods, but also, as anthropologist Robert Ranulph Marett tells us, "a higher plane of
experience . . . in which spiritual enlargement is appreciated for its own sake." In
this book, we are concerned with this spiritual enlargement (the expansion process)
as well as with the healing and transformative properties of crystals.

Using This Book

So many new crystals are entering the market today that it can be hard to keep
up—or to know which ones will be really useful. In this book, you will find stones
revered for more than ten thousand years, as well as some newly discovered ones.

Each is attributed a specific power that sums up its overall effect, but I offer
a broader description of its healing and transformational properties as well. You'll
find crystals for love, health, protection, abundance, longevity, justice, and more.
Not all crystals suit everyone, so my selection offers alternatives and new possibilities to resonate with your unique energy field. I also explain how to harness each
crystal's power. Once you become accustomed to working with crystals, you can
apply these techniques to your other crystals.

The chakra diagram with information (page 14) can further assist you in working with stones. A glossary starting on page 216 explains terms with which you may
be unfamiliar. Instructions for choosing appropriate crystals, as well as purifying,
activating, and maintaining their powers, are given on pages 10–13.

High-Vibration Crystals

Some crystals, such as Selenite and Danburite, already possessed a light, high vibration that activates the higher chakras. But new finds of Danburite and other well-known crystals that have a higher-vibration of the basic power have become available. For example, natural Golden Danburite (Agni Gold™) and the alchemicalized Aqua Aura Danburite have the underlying properties of the basic Danburite crystal, but raise these to another dimension.

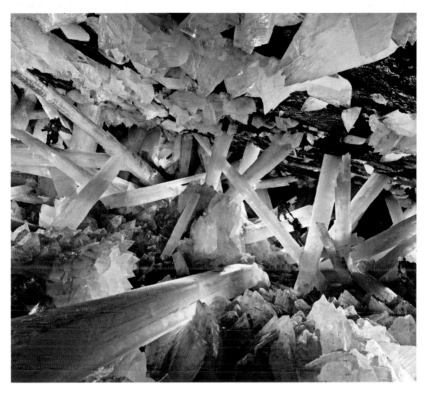

These enormous Selenite crystals grow in a Mexican cavern so hot that human beings in fire-protection gear can only stay for a few minutes.

Some completely new high-vibration stones, along with extremely high-vibration varieties of Quartz now on the market, also assist in raising consciousness. These resonate with the high-vibration chakras that connect us to greater realities (see page 14). High-vibration crystals and their associated chakras facilitate the expansion process, an evolution and extension of your awareness to encompass the multidimensions of spiritual life.

How to Find the Right Crystal for You

Seek not to measure the material, but consider rather the power which reason has and mere substance not.— Manilius (Roman astrologer)

Finding the right stone for you is the key to attuning yourself to crystal power. You'll probably start by searching for a crystal that holds the power you want to manifest. Or, one of the stunning pictures in this book might catch your eye. But where do you go from here? What if you have no idea which crystal is right for you?

Use your own magical power of attraction! Put out the focused thought: "I find exactly the right crystal for me, now." Go into a store and run your hands through a basket of crystals. One will "stick" to your fingers, or you'll relish the feel as you pick one up. This is the crystal for you. You may already have the right stone in your collection. Wherever you find your crystal, make sure you purify and empower it before use. When choosing a crystal, remember the biggest and flashiest is not necessarily the best for your purpose. The Roman poet Claudian offered an adage wise crystal workers still use today:

> *Pass not the shapeless lump of crystal by*
> *Nor view the icy mass with careless eye . . .*
> *This rough and unform'd stone, without a grace,*
> *Midst rarest treasures holds the chiefest place.*

It is not the outward beauty of a crystal that indicates its power, but rather what it does for you. A rough lump of raw rock may be more powerful than a faceted gemstone, no matter how seductive the latter may be.

Crystal Attunement

Take a few moments to attune to a crystal. Hold a purified crystal in your hands and feel its vibrations radiating into your being. If they are in accord with your own, you will feel calm, peaceful, and quite possibly expanded. If you feel uncomfortable, choose another stone—the one you are holding might not be right for you at this time, or may indicate you have inner work to do.

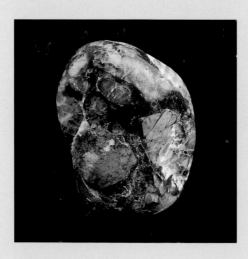

The Power of Shape

Crystals naturally possess internal and external geometric shapes, which mold how energy flows through them. But many crystals are artificially shaped externally to enhance their power flow. Knowing how the external shape enhances the power helps you select the right crystal for your purpose.

Take Amethyst, for example. You'll find Amethyst in cavelike geodes, single points, clusters, beds, balls, and palm stones. All carry Amethyst's underlying peace of mind, but how that power radiates varies according to the stone's shape.

GEODE

The cavelike interior of a geode collects, amplifies, and stores crystal power, and then gently radiates it out to the environment. It provides protection, creates abundance, and encourages spiritual growth. In *Natural History*, Pliny says that geodes treat eyes, breasts, and testicles, an example of a shared shape or "sympathy" between the crystal and the area being healed.

POINT

Points, including wands, focus crystal power into a single concentrated beam. When you place the point toward your body, it channels power into your body. Aim the point out and it draws off negative energy.

PHANTOM

Phantom crystals are laid down in layers, often pyramidal in shape, within another type of crystal. Holding the memory of the soul's journey, they break up ancient patterns of behavior or can be ascended like a ladder to higher consciousness.

CLUSTER

Clusters are a group of points radiating out in different directions. They beam energy into the surrounding atmosphere, but can also be empowered to draw off negative energy.

BED

A bed has many small crystals spread over a matrix base. This provides a steady source of crystal power, like a battery does. Beds are particularly useful when you need continuous crystal power.

BALL

Balls are artificially shaped from a larger piece of crystal; they emit power in all directions in equal measure. Balls provide a focus for powers such as insight or intuition. Traditionally, crystal balls were used to see forward or backward in time, a practice known as scrying.

PALM STONE

Flat and rounded, palm stones are tactile reminders of crystal power. Holding one soothes the mind, so you focus intention to create what you desire.

MANIFESTATION

This crystal has a smaller crystal encased within the main one. As its name suggests, it carries the power of manifestation—especially of abundance—but can be harnessed to any crystal power.

Maintaining Crystal Power

Crystals must be purified and activated to bring their power to life—and they must be kept cleansed to maintain that power. It is no good buying a crystal, putting it in your pocket, and expecting it to work miracles—unless you've asked it to. As a first step, as Shakespeare, who knew of the esoteric power of stones, instructs in *Henry V*, "Go, clear thy crystals." Once you've purified your crystal, its power can be dedicated to your highest good.

Treat your crystals with respect and work with them in partnership. They will repay you with years of devoted service. Treat them badly or misuse them, and their power may turn against you. They are, after all, magical, sentient beings.

RIGHT USE OF POWER

Crystals work by cooperating with you to focus and manifest your intention. Be clear about why you are working with the crystal and ensure that you are working for the highest good. Misuse of crystal power will inevitably rebound. Like humans, crystals can become exhausted, so re-empowering them regularly is a sensible precaution. As crystals rapidly draw off energy from their surroundings, they need purifying at frequent intervals.

PURIFYING YOUR CRYSTALS

Crystals pick up energy from anyone who handles them and from the environment, so they need cleansing before and after use. Purify a crystal by holding it under running water—so long as the crystal won't dissolve or fragment. Then put it in the sun or moonlight to reenergize it. You can also smudge a crystal with incense smoke, place it in candlelight, or leave it overnight in uncooked brown rice.

ACTIVATING THE POWER OF YOUR CRYSTAL

To activate your crystal's power, hold the purified crystal in your hands, focus your intention and attention on it, and say:

> *"I dedicate this crystal to the highest good of all*
> *and ask that its power be activated now to work in harmony*
> *with my own will and focused intention."*

If you have a specific purpose, add that to your dedication. To deactivate the crystal, cleanse it and then hold the crystal as you say:

> *"I thank this crystal for its power, which is no longer needed at this time.*
> *I ask that its power be closed until reactivated."*

Put the crystal in the sun to recharge it, and then place it in a bag, box, or a drawer until it is required again.

If you are placing crystals in a grid, layout for cleaning, or to create safe space, join up the shape either by touching each stone with a crystal wand or by using the power of your mind to picture lines of light connecting the stones and making the shape.

Using Crystal Power

After you have empowered your crystal, you can wear it daily, preferably in contact with your skin. Or, place it on your body or in your environment to radiate out or draw on the power as appropriate. A piece of Black Tourmaline or Amber, for instance, placed in each corner of your home invokes the power of protection and energy screening, safeguarding you. Or, you can use your crystal for healing or to expand your consciousness.

One of the easiest ways to tap into a crystal's healing power is to place the crystal over an appropriate chakra or organ for fifteen minutes to rebalance the energy center. The crystal descriptions in this book give physiological and chakra connections. Regular cleansing and reenergizing of your chakras (the body's psychic immune system) maintains your energy at optimum levels and stimulates your personal power.

If a crystal produces a healing challenge (an intensification of "symptoms"), remove it and put Smoky Quartz in its place. You can also reharmonize the subtle nervous system with Natrolite or Scolecite (see pages 134).

To expand your consciousness with high-vibration crystals, either place a crystal on your third eye, soma, or higher crown chakra, or sit holding the stone. Breathe gently and focus your awareness on the crystal. Do not try to see or experience anything, simply let the process unfold. Notice any changes, without giving them undue attention.

After ten to twenty minutes (no longer), remove the crystal. Picture yourself totally surrounded by a bubble of crystal light. Feel the contact your feet make with the Earth, and then get up and go about your everyday business. If you feel "floaty" or unfocused, hold a Smoky Quartz or Hematite as you visualize roots growing from the balls of your feet, joining at the earth star chakra, and then going down into the center of the Earth where they attach to the ball of iron at its center to create a shamanic anchor.

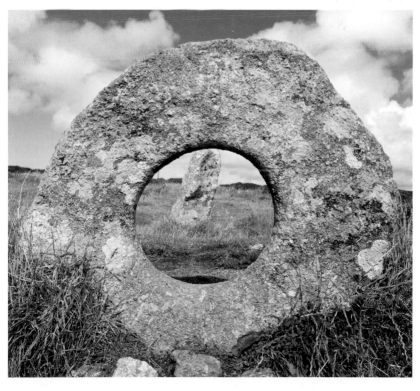

Men-an-Tol alignment, Cornwall. Since ancient times, the sick have been passed through this granite holed stone as a traditional form of healing.

Chakra Power

Each chakra powers a sphere of life. Imbalances can cause physical dis-ease as well as specific personality traits and issues that can be healed with crystals:

Chakra diagram

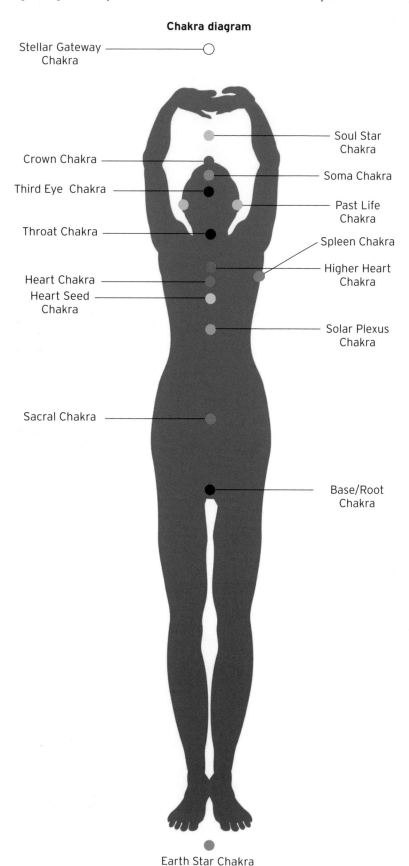

Stellar Gateway Chakra

Soul Star Chakra

Crown Chakra

Soma Chakra

Third Eye Chakra

Past Life Chakra

Throat Chakra

Spleen Chakra

Higher Heart Chakra

Heart Chakra

Heart Seed Chakra

Solar Plexus Chakra

Sacral Chakra

Base/Root Chakra

Earth Star Chakra

EARTH STAR CHAKRA

Key issues: Everyday reality and groundedness. Picks up adverse environmental factors, such as geopathic stress and toxic pollutants. Imbalances or blockages lead to physical discomfort, feeling of helplessness, and inability to function practically.

Negative power: powerlessness

Positive power: empowerment

Dis-eases are lethargic: myalgic encephalomyelitis (ME), arthritis, cancer, muscular disorders, depression, psychiatric disturbances, autoimmune diseases

BASE/ROOT CHAKRA

Key issues: Basic survival instincts and security. Triggers the fight-or-flight response. Imbalances lead to sexual disturbances and feelings of being stuck, anger, impotence, frustration, and inability to let go.

Negative power: insecurity and alienation

Positive power: inner security and connectedness

Dis-eases are constant and low-level, or flare up suddenly: stiffness in joints; chronic lower back pain; renal, reproductive, or rectal disorders; fluid retention; constipation (diarrhea if stuck open); varicose veins or hernias; bipolar disorder; glandular disturbances; personality and anxiety disorders; autoimmune diseases

SACRAL CHAKRA

Key issues: Creativity, fertility, acceptance of yourself as a powerful and sexual being. "Hooks" from other people make themselves felt, particularly from previous sexual encounters. Imbalances lead to infertility and blocked creativity.

Negative power: selfishness with low self-esteem

Positive power: self-worth, confidence

Dis-eases are toxic and psychosomatic: PMS, muscle cramps, reproductive blockages or diseases, impotence, infertility, allergies, addictions, eating disorders, diabetes, liver or intestinal dysfunction, irritable bowel, chronic back pain, urinary infections

SOLAR PLEXUS CHAKRA

Key issues: Emotional processing and communication. Energy assimilation and utilization, concentration. Emotional "hooks" from other people are found here. "Illness as theater" plays out the emotional story through life circumstances. Blockages lead to being overwhelmed by emotions or taking on other people's feelings and problems.

Negative power: inferiority, clinginess

Positive power: emotional stability

Dis-eases are emotional and demanding: stomach ulcers, ME, adrenaline imbalances, insomnia, chronic anxiety, digestive problems, gallstones, pancreatic failure, eczema and other skin conditions, eating disorders, phobias

HEART SEED CHAKRA

Key issues: Soul remembrance and universal love. If blocked, spiritual purpose is lost.

Negative power: rootlessness and disconnection

Positive power: awareness of purpose of incarnation and connection to divine plan

Dis-eases are psycho-spiritual, not physical.

HEART CHAKRA

Key issues: Love and nurturance. If blocked, love cannot flourish. Feelings such as jealousy are common with enormous resistance to change.

Negative power: possessiveness

Positive power: compassion and peaceful harmony

Dis-eases are psychosomatic and reactive: heart attacks, angina, chest infections, asthma, frozen shoulder, ulcers

SPLEEN CHAKRA

Key issues: Assertion and empowerment. Psychic vampires link in here to get their energy fix. Imbalances cause anger issues or constant irritation; the body attacks itself. If too open, other people draw on your energy, causing depletion at immune level.

Negative power: aggression

Positive power: self-assertiveness and empowerment

Dis-eases arise from depletion: lethargy, anemia, low blood sugar

HIGHER HEART CHAKRA (THYMUS)

Key issues: Compassion. Blockages cause emotional neediness and inability to express feelings openly; unconditional love and service cannot be offered.

Negative power: neediness

Positive power: unconditional love

Dis-eases of the heart and immune deficiencies: arteriosclerosis, viral infections, tinnitus, epilepsy

THROAT CHAKRA

Key issues: Communication. If blocked, thoughts and feelings cannot be verbalized nor truth expressed. Other people's opinions can cause difficulties.

Negative power: mendacity

Positive power: truthful self-expression

Dis-eases relate to root beliefs, are active, and block communication: sore throat/quinsy, inflammation of trachea, sinus, constant colds, viral infections, tinnitus and ear infections, jaw pain, gum disease, tooth problems, thyroid imbalances, high blood pressure, ADHD, autism, speech impediment, and psychosomatic dis-eases such as irritable bowel

THIRD EYE CHAKRA

Key issues: Intuition and mental connection. Imbalances allow bombardment by other people's thoughts, or wild and irrational intuitions. Other people's control, beliefs, or coercing mental "hooks" affect thoughts.

Negative power: delusion

Positive power: intuitive insight

Dis-eases are intuitive and metaphysical: migraines, mental overwhelm, schizophrenia, cataracts, iritis and eye problems, epilepsy, autism, spinal and neurological disorders, sinus and ear infections, high blood pressure, irritations of all kinds

PAST LIFE CHAKRA

Key issues: Memory and hereditary issues. Imbalances keep you stuck in the past; you cannot move forward, repeating personal past-life patterns or ancestral patterns passed through the family. People from the past attach to and control you.

Negative power: dependence

Positive power: self-direction

Dis-eases are chronic and reflect previous wounds: immune or endocrine deficiencies, and genetic, neurotransmitter or physical malfunctions.

SOMA CHAKRA

Key issues: Spiritual identity, expansion, soul journeying. Imbalances create disembodied "airheads" with little connection to the physical world or their physical bodies; or overly strong embodiedness traps the soul and prevents spiritual connection.

Negative power: disconnection from material or spiritual world

Positive power: awareness of being both physically in incarnation and spiritually expanded

Dis-eases are autistic and disconnected or dyspraxic and may include Down syndrome.

CROWN CHAKRA

Key issues: Spiritual communication and awareness. If blocked, you may attempt to control others; if stuck open, obsession and openness to spiritual interference or possession can occur. When imbalanced, excessive environmental sensitivity and delusions or dementia result.

Negative power: arrogance

Positive power: spirituality

Dis-eases arise from disconnection: metabolic syndrome, illness with no known cause, nervous system disturbances, electromagnetic and environmental sensitivity, depression, dementia, ME, insomnia or excessive sleepiness, biological clock disturbances

SOUL STAR CHAKRA

Key issues: Soul connection and spiritual illumination. If blocked or stuck open, soul fragmentation occurs; messiah complex or openness to invasion from "alien" entities may occur.

Negative power: disconnected and spiritual arrogance

Positive power: enlightenment

Dis-eases are spiritual, not physical.

STELLAR GATEWAY CHAKRA

Key issues: Cosmic portal. If blocked or stuck open, contacts with low-level entities and dissemination of spiritual misinformation can occur.

Negative power: delusions

Positive power: cosmic consciousness

Dis-eases are spiritual, not physical.

Scepter

- **Chakra correspondences:** Ignites and empowers all chakras, particularly the base and sacral
- **Physiological correspondences:** Male genitalia, female reproductive system, endocrine glands
- **Vibration:** Earthy to high depending on the particular type of crystal (a Scepter is a specific shape, not a type of crystal)

LEGENDARY POWER

The ultimate symbol of power, Scepter is a shape rather than a specific type of crystal. It can be likened to a magician's wand. A Scepter's central rod has another crystal—usually, but not always, of the same type—wrapped around it. Its shape may be phallic/masculine or yonic/feminine. A reversed Scepter has a small crystal point emerging from a larger base. Scepters may be naturally formed or carved from a piece of crystal.

An ancient symbol of royal authority, the Scepter also formed part of priestly regalia. As most early priests and kings were shamans and magicians, the Scepter took on an aura of awesome power. In the Greek *Iliad* (ninth century B.C.E.), Homer speaks of a Scepter made from a wooden rod topped with an ornamented ball, the whole overlaid in gold and adorned with precious stones. Virtually all the European countries include a Scepter among ceremonial regalia, symbolizing the monarch's inalienable right to rule.

HEALING POWER

A Scepter directs healing energy precisely to the source of a problem in the physical or subtle bodies, so that energies are restructured and brought into alignment. The shape magnifies the innate healing power of the crystal and dissolves or blasts out sources of dis-ease, depending on the crystal's nature. A Malachite or Obsidian Scepter, for instance, produces a powerful blast of energy, whereas an Amethyst or Elestial is gentler in its approach.

A Scepter is particularly helpful in dealing with the emotional and psychological impact of childhood abuse where this is an underlying psychosomatic cause of dis-ease. In past-life work, a Scepter helps to heal personality splits created by soul or karmic wounds, especially if these have been caused by an abuse of authority. A Scepter also assists in reintegrating soul fragments. The shape unites masculine and feminine energies to stimulate the controlled rise of kundalini power to activate enlightenment.

TRANSFORMATIONAL POWER

All Scepters assist you with assimilating and using power properly. An Elestial Quartz Scepter is the ultimate tool for reclaiming lost power, whether power was willingly handed over or has been lost through abuse or misuse of power in the past. It is especially useful if this loss of power has caused psychological dis-ease, anxiety, and personality disorders. Calling your power back transforms you into an inner-directed being who cannot be swayed by external influences. You are empowered.

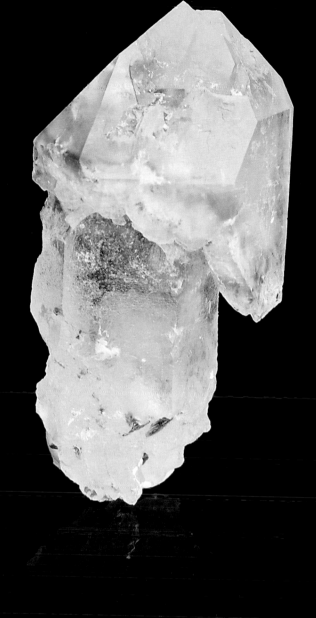

To activate your power, place
the Scepter over your base chakra
for five minutes and say aloud:
"I reclaim and activate my
power now."

Agate

- **Chakra correspondences:** Varies according to color and type; stabilizes and cleanses all chakras
- **Physiological correspondences:** Skin, eyes, lymphatic system and fluid balance, uterus, stomach and digestive processes, blood vessels, pancreas, skin, emotional balance, mental concentration
- **Vibration:** Earthy

LEGENDARY POWER

Agate symbolizes wealth, health, and longevity. In Mesopotamia, Agates were engraved as seal stones (symbols of power and authority). Pliny wrote that the Romans used the stone to make mortar and pestles with which to grind medicines.

Agate supports life in difficult circumstances, keeping the soul from harm. Legend said that eagles carried Agates to their nests to protect their young from snakebites, so early people wore Agate amulets to guard against the venomous bites of spiders or scorpions. In China, Agate was believed to be the solidified blood of the ancestors. In India and North Africa, red Agates were thought to contain the blood of demons and thus afforded protection against evil spirits.

Agate is associated with Archangel Michael and the Shekinah, the divine feminine and merciful Queen of Heaven who rules karmic release, wholeness, and blessings. Almost certainly in the biblical Breastplate of the High Priest, Agate would have been the eighth stone, connecting it to Scorpio.

HEALING POWER

Travelers in the Arabian and African deserts sucked Agates to overcome the effects of thirst. In the Middle Ages, the stones were used to heal dropsy and fever, relieve insomnia, firm the gums, and prevent epilepsy in children. Today, crystal workers harness Agate's power to bring stability to the physical body and aura, cleanse the lymphatic system, and regulate fluid balance. The stone assists emotional healing and strengthens mental concentration.

TRANSFORMATIONAL POWER

Agate puts you in touch with your inner self. Its power lies in its ability to transmute dark, toxic emotions such as jealousy, bitterness, and resentment, which have a psychosomatic effect on the body, creating dis-ease in the heart and unrest in the soul. Due to its powerful cleansing effect, Agate helps you assimilate challenging life experiences and recognize the spiritual gifts they offer. By promoting self-acceptance and forgiveness, Agate increases receptivity to spiritual currents in your life. Carrying an Agate stimulates courage to start again and encourages you to hold fast to your own truth. It helps you recognize your eternal nature and the oneness of all things.

Although some Agates feature brilliant colors, these effects are created by humans, not nature. The raw stones are heated with minerals, such as iron, to turn dull slices of rock into rainbows of color. Agate reminds us that no matter how base the material we start with, it can be tempered and transformed by spiritual alchemy.

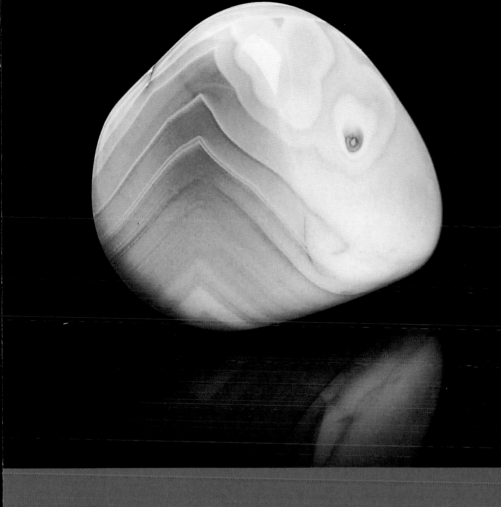

Wear Agate or keep one in your
pocket and touch it frequently
to give you strength.

Ajoite

- **Chakra correspondences:** Third eye, crown, soma, soul star, stellar gateway; links the soul star, heart, and throat chakras
- **Physiological correspondences:** Cellular structures and cellular memory, immune system
- **Vibration:** Exceptionally high

LEGENDARY POWER

Ajoite was named after Ajo in Arizona. Modern crystal lore considers Ajoite one of the most important stones for high-vibration work and powering the shift to the Aquarian Age. Used as a vibrational runway to expanded consciousness and spiritual awakening, Ajoite facilitates expanded consciousness so rapidly it can feel like a spaceship blasting into orbit.

Paradoxically, though, Ajoite reminds you that spiritual evolution has to take place on the Earth. This stone helps you feel at home on our planet. In Arkansas, Ajoite is found in combination with Shattuckite crystal and Calcite, creating powerful synergistic protection and acceleration for the soul's journey.

HEALING POWER

Ajoite cleanses the auric field, especially the emotional body, and aligns it with the higher chakras in preparation for expansion. This crystal induces profound calm, and helps you release stress and anxiety. Most of Ajoite's healing power lies in its ability to facilitate reunion with the divine. Although mainly a stone for experienced crystal workers to use, novices can place it in bathwater to gently transfer its energy to your physical and subtle bodies, and to attune you to higher vibrations. Extremely effective for harmonizing the physical body with a realigned etheric blueprint and for stimulating cellular memory, this crystal awakens higher DNA patterns. It stabilizes cell structures and the subtle immune system to a new vibration. Ajoite facilitates karmic healing and removes energetic implants from the body, no matter what their source.

TRANSFORMATIONAL POWER

The gentle energies of Ajoite draw out from the physical, emotional, mental, and spiritual bodies any toxic emotions, thoughts, beliefs, constructs, or blockages that have prevented an influx of higher energies, thereby enabling your whole being to evolve spiritually. Its vibration teaches the value of forgiving and accepting yourself and others. If you have been carrying a burden or felt an overwhelming, inappropriate responsibility for someone else, Ajoite helps you detach and allow the other person to follow his or her own path. This stone also shows you what your true higher purpose and path are. Ajoite opens the soma chakra to allow the energy body and the soul to journey through multiple dimensions. Because it holds the vibration of infinite compassion, Ajoite enfolds the soul in unconditional, universal love and promotes connection with the angelic realms. Ajoite is perfect for timid people who want to reach multidimensional consciousness and become awakened beings.

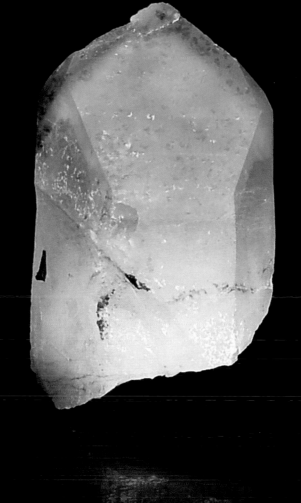

Meditate with Ajoite,
held to your third eye or soma
chakra, to open and expand your
spiritual awareness.

Amazonite

- **Chakra correspondences:** Spleen, solar plexus, heart, throat; opens and stabilizes all chakras
- **Physiological correspondences:** Spleen, metabolic processes, thyroid and parathyroid glands, liver, bones, teeth, nervous system, calcium utilization, muscles
- **Vibration:** Earthy; brilliant turquoise Amazonite has a higher vibration than green

LEGENDARY POWER

Greek mythology chronicles the Amazons, a matriarchal tribe of women warriors who worshipped Artemis, virgin goddess of the hunt, wild places, and the moon. Artemis was "virgin" because she integrated masculine and feminine energies and was intact psychologically, rather than in the physical sense. The Greeks believed the Amazons inhabited a mysterious space between the known and unknown worlds.

These warlike women were a close-knit sisterhood that valued friendship, courage, and loyalty. Amazons cut off their right breasts, directing all their strength into their right arms so they could better draw their bows. These independent women mated only when necessary for the survival of the race, directing their reproductive and creative energies into the arts of war and sisterhood.

Amazonite was named after the Amazon River rather than the tribe, but the stone carries many Amazonian attributes, including strength, fortitude, and the power of friendship. It helps you integrate masculine and feminine energies and assists you in seeing both sides of a problem before seeking resolution.

HEALING POWER

Amazonite shields the body from the effects of subtle radiation and electromagnetic frequencies, including Wi-Fi, which depletes the immune systems in sensitive people. The stone also aligns the subtle nervous system with the physical nervous system and may relieve muscle spasm. Because Amazonite resonates with calcium, crystal workers use it to regulate calcium uptake in the body and to balance metabolic deficiencies that create osteoporosis, tooth decay, and calcification.

TRANSFORMATIONAL POWER

The green coloring of Amazonite comes from traces of lead, which may explain why, according to the principles of sympathetic magic, it is an effective shield against electromagnetic smog. The stone transforms consequent dis-ease into optimum well-being.

Amazonite transmutes destructive emotional patterns and deconstructs ingrained beliefs, encouraging creative thinking to help you consciously create a new reality. It assists women who have been unable to have children to find other outlets for their creative energy, and helps those who suffer from "empty nest syndrome" redirect their nurturing abilities. If you need courage to move forward in life and break codependent tendencies, Amazonite encourages independence while drawing supportive friends to you.

Brilliant turquoise Amazonite has a finer energetic frequency than green. It provides powerful protection when you are exploring the higher realms of consciousness. It disentangles detrimental karmic connections that operate through the higher chakras, freeing your soul energies and reconnecting you to your proper soul group.

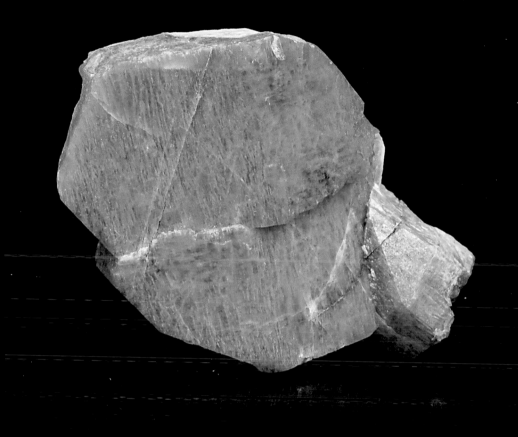

HARNESSING THE POWER

To share the power of friendship,
give your friends Amazonites.
Schedule a regular time when you
will think of each other while
holding your stones.

Amber

- **Chakra correspondences:** Sacral, throat, higher heart (thymus); cleanses all chakras
- **Physiological correspondences:** Throat, joints, mucus membranes, liver, gallbladder, kidneys, spleen, stomach, immune system
- **Vibration:** Earthy, but protects in higher dimensions

LEGENDARY POWER

Amber has long been associated with protection and renewal, in part because the insects perfectly preserved within it look as though they could spring to life and fly away at any moment. These inclusions led to Amber's reputation as the repository of departed souls.

Theophrastus pointed out that Amber attracts iron, a reference to its electrostatic properties. When rubbed against skin, silk, or wool, Amber becomes electrically charged—paper and feathers stick to it. This must have appeared magical indeed, leading Aristotle to credit the resin with having a soul. Pliny mentions that Amber was created by moisture from the rays of the sun falling upon the Earth, and was associated with the sun's life-giving energy.

HEALING POWER

Amber ignites easily, and the ancients believed its smoke drove away evil spirits and enchantments, as well as relieving sinus and respiratory ailments and throat infections. Pliny attributed to Amber the powers of healing blindness and "affectations of the ears," as well as curing fevers. Ground into a powder and mixed with honey or oil, Amber was used in Europe, Egypt, and Arabia as a natural antibiotic for healing wounds and regenerating tissue. Believed to be a remedy against plague, goiter, epilepsy, jaundice, rheumatism, and heart disease, it allegedly changed color in the presence of poison. The handles of ancient Jewish and Arabic circumcision and surgical knives were carved from Amber as it was thought to staunch bleeding.

Amber's power stimulates the body's natural healing mechanisms. Modern crystal healers place Amber over a wound to promote healing or at the thymus gland to restore balance to the body.

TRANSFORMATIONAL POWER

Amber can be used to transmute negative vibrations into positive ones. It creates an efficient screen against negative energies of all kinds. Placed on the body, it energetically cleanses and reactivates the chakras and your psychic immune system. Put Amber in the corners of a sickroom to keep it energetically clean and to shield the patient against adverse environmental energies.

If you lack the drive to succeed, Amber motivates you to make decisions and move forward in life. It helps you transmute dreams into practical reality. With its assistance, you recognize true worth in yourself and others, as Amber indicates disdain for those who prize wealth above personal quality.

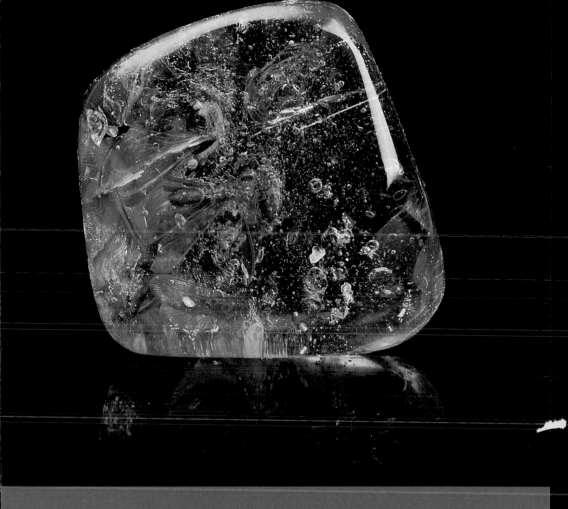

Hold a piece of Amber above
your head and imagine it slowly
melting, pouring a protective
coating around your aura to seal it.

Amethyst

- **Chakra correspondences:** Third eye, crown, soma, soul star, stellar gateway, and beyond
- **Physiological correspondences:** Cellular and metabolic processes, endocrine function, hormone regulation, neural transmission, brain harmonization, immune system, blood, skin, respiratory and digestive tracts, skin, psychosomatic disorders
- **Vibration:** High (Vera Cruz, Brandenberg, Amethyst Elestial, and Sirius Amethyst have exceptionally high vibrations)

LEGENDARY POWER

Amethyst means "sincerity" and "freedom from harm." Symbolizing wisdom, deep love, devotion, and peace of mind, the stone was worn historically by royalty to signify power. Amethyst's legendary power protected against drunkenness—the name literally means "not drunk." Ancient Romans drank wine from amethyst cups, and for millennia people wore Amethysts to prevent intoxication.

Amethyst's color comes from iron, but according to Greek mythology, the god of wine, Bacchus, was offended by Diana, the huntress. In revenge, he declared that the first person he met in the forest would be eaten by his tiger. A beautiful maiden called Amethyst was on her way to worship at the shrine of Diana when she met the tiger. Calling on the goddess to save her, she turned into a sparkling white crystal. Repenting, Bacchus poured wine over her, producing the stone's characteristic purple hue.

Amethyst is one of the stones in the Breastplate of the High Priest and a stone for Archangel Raphael. It is worn in the Christian church to signify high rank, victory over worldly passion, and spiritual power. According to the eighth-century Archbishop of Mainz, Amethyst instills in humble souls the constant thought of heaven.

HEALING POWER

Amethyst's vibrations remove subtle dis-ease. An effective tranquilizer, it helps you understand the source of addictions. Traditionally, Amethyst was bound to the forehead to heal headaches, and modern-day crystal workers use Amethyst to calm anxiety and draw off physical or psychological pain. It balances the subtle endocrine system, regulating hormone production. The stone may aid psychosomatic diseases of the digestive tract by transmuting whatever is, metaphorically, hard to swallow. It reduces swelling anywhere on the body.

An Amethyst geode or cluster is an excellent tool for space clearing or Earth healing, as it absorbs negativity and infuses an area with tranquility. Amethyst blocks geopathic stress and electromagnetic frequencies.

TRANSFORMATIONAL POWER

Amethyst opens your third eye and clarifies spiritual vision. By creating a safe sacred space for meditation and multidimensional exploration, it clears your mind and aids enlightenment. High-vibration Amethysts, such as Vera Cruz, act on an altogether different level. Placed on the soul star or stellar gateway chakra, they stimulate your soul to remember its origins and facilitate multidimensional cellular healing. By detaching you from unwanted entities, thought forms, or mental constructs, Amethyst dispels illusions that prevent you from experiencing true reality. It helps you dream a new world into being.

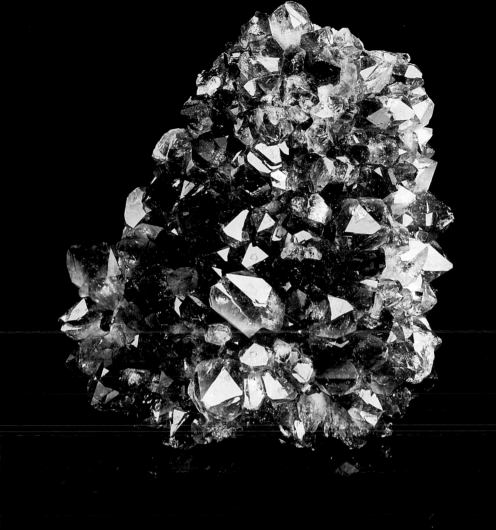

Place an Amethyst above
your head, point toward you,
and one on your forehead,
pointing down. Feel peace
radiating through your body.

Amphibole Quartz

- **Chakra correspondences:** Stellar gateway, soul star, third eye, crown, soma, higher heart (thymus)
- **Physiological correspondences:** Immune system; this crystal functions at the subtle and spiritual levels rather than the physical
- **Vibration:** Exceptionally high

LEGENDARY POWER

Modern crystal lore credits Amphibole Quartz with having an angelic presence. Synonymous with Archangel Gabriel, Amphibole can be used to call in guardian angels and higher beings. Angels are vast energetic force fields with rapidly oscillating frequencies that enable them to traverse multiple dimensions, rather than the anthropomorphic beings usually pictured. They can, however, appear in any guise when interacting with humans.

The Jewish Old Testament, Apocrypha, Christian New Testament, Koran, and many older writings, such as the Mesopotamia creation myths, chronicle encounters with angels. Throughout these and other cultures, angels and winged beings have intervened in human affairs, offering guidance, protection, and healing. Amphibole Quartz lets you perceive the presence of angels and attune yourself to divine emanations. It stimulates the mental body and raises the frequency of the brain's central cortex to prepare it for an influx of universal consciousness.

HEALING POWER

Amphibole Quartz functions at a high vibratory level to bring the subtle bodies into harmony and activate intuitive rebalancing of the soul body. Holding the crystal acts as a first aid measure when you feel out of sorts or display symptoms of dis-ease, as it quickly restores well-being. The stone's vibrations energetically heal space, infusing it with peace and love, harmonizing it to the highest possible vibration to ensure cooperation within that space. It is the perfect carrier for etheric-cleansing essences as it holds a vibration and radiates it out for several days.

TRANSFORMATIONAL POWER

Hold Amphibole Quartz to fill your body with profound joy. It contains Hematite, which grounds and stabilizes higher forces; Limonite, which guards against psychic attack and undue mental influences; and Kaolinite, which opens the inner ear so you hear the voice of your intuition. Amphibole Quartz helps break up old patterns and reconnects you to the wisdom of your soul. A perfect crystal for spiritual journeying and exploring higher dimensions, Amphibole Quartz takes you into the heart of universal love. Tuck one into your pocket to ensure that you always walk in the presence of angels. If you are an angel who has assumed physical form to assist humanity's spiritual evolution, this crystal's power helps you recognize the totality of your angelic being.

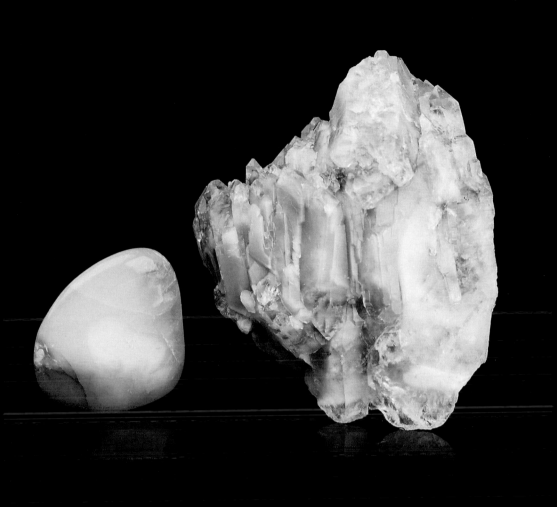

To call in your guardian angel or
to petition angelic guidance, sleep
with Amphibole under your pillow.

Apatite

- **Chakra correspondences:** Third eye, base, solar plexus; harmonizes all
- **Physiological correspondences:** Nervous, endocrine, and metabolic systems; biological clock; brain function; bones; teeth; cartilage; joints; thyroid; parathyroid; motor function; cellular structures; regeneration; calcium absorption; kundalini; hyperactivity; blood pressure; detoxification; liver; gallbladder; spleen; mental subtle body
- **Vibration:** Earthy to high, depending on color

LEGENDARY POWER

Apatite has a reputation as a mystical crystal and is valued for its ability to stimulate metaphysical abilities and orchestrate the subtle metabolic system via the chakras. It stimulates the pineal, which the philosopher Descartes called the seat of the soul. When your pineal is fully activated, you experience what William Blake called "the world in a grain of sand and eternity in an hour."

It is postulated that the pineal secretes DMT, the "spirit molecule." A neurochemical looking glass, DMT is a natural psychedelic involved in out-of-body, near-death, and other Exceptional Human Experiences (EHEs).

HEALING POWER

Calcium-rich Apatite contains a mineral naturally produced in the body: hydroxylapatite. A major component of bones and tooth enamel, hydroxylapatite is found in the "brain sand" present in the pineal, which produces the melatonin that regulates biorhythms and circadian cycles. The pineal has also been shown to monitor the effects of electromagnetic fields and to regulate the body accordingly.

Crystal workers heal metabolic disturbances and dis-eases created by calcium imbalances with Apatite. An accumulation of fluorite in the pineal gland has a detrimental effect on sleep patterns, as well as on puberty and sexual maturation. Under the principle of "like heals like," Apatite energetically releases excess fluoride and calcium. It may dissolve concretions and rebalance bone-building, cellular, and metabolic processes. Apatite may also reduce hypertension caused by an overabundance of calcium in the body. Position this crystal over joints to assist cartilage and bone development or to ease muscle pain. Held against the cheek near the teeth, it encourages good dentition. Additionally, Apatite contains phosphorus, the second-most abundant mineral in the body. Phosphorus is required for genetic building-block function, healthy nerve tissue, bone growth, filtration of waste from the kidneys, and correct storage and utilization of energy.

Crystal lore says Apatite confers immortality as it aids the elimination of free radicals, slowing the aging process. By reducing wrinkles, it is said to make you look younger. Placed on the crown chakra, Apatite balances the brain's hemispheres, harnessing left- and right-brain perception modes and stimulating neurotransmitters.

TRANSFORMATIONAL POWER

This inspirational crystal works at the energetic interface between matter and consciousness, an interface reflected in the pineal gland with its powerful connection to the spiritual and metaphysical worlds. Put Yellow or rarer Purple Apatite on the soma and crown chakras to awaken spiritually.

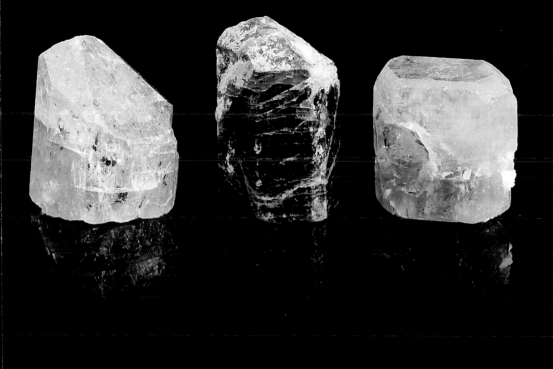

Place Blue Apatite on your third
eye and Yellow Apatite on your
crown chakra to accelerate your
rational mind and integrate mental
and intuitive abilities.

Apophyllite

- **Chakra correspondences:** Third eye, soma, crown, soul star, stellar gateway, heart, heart seed
- **Physiological correspondences:** Eyes, skin, respiratory system, mucus membranes
- **Vibration:** High to very high

LEGENDARY POWER

Apophyllite brings illumination and clarity to any situation, material or spiritual. The perfect crystal for self-attunement, Apophyllite is a combination of three minerals that stimulate the pineal gland and open inner sight. Traditionally used for enhancing metaphysical abilities, such as clairvoyance and telepathy, Apophyllite pyramids and mirrors make excellent scrying tools when looked into obliquely from the corner of the eye rather than directly. Place an Apophyllite pyramid on your third eye to facilitate mental clarity, calm your mind, and remove confusion. It also helps you develop channeling or kything abilities.

When positioned on the soma chakra, Apophyllite stimulates safe out-of-body journeying, keeping the connection between the physical and subtle bodies strong. Placed on the third eye or past life chakra, Apophyllite lets you read the Akashic Record, the cosmic account of all that has been and will occur. It can take you back into the past for karmic healing or into the future to assess the outcome of the choices you make now. This crystal promotes total honesty and harmony with the people around you.

HEALING POWER

Apophyllite works best at a subtle level to heal the spirit and help your soul come to terms with being incarnated. With the assistance of Apophyllite, you learn to pay attention to the needs of your physical body and your soul, preventing psychosomatic and soul-based illnesses from taking root. In its pyramid form, Apophyllite focuses healing energy into a beam that can break up energetic blockages, draw off negative energy, and replace them with healing light.

Placed on the chest, Apophyllite may relieve asthma attacks caused by allergies. Due to its high water content, the crystal energetically rehydrates mucus membranes in your respiratory tract and eyes. Apophyllite enhances the flow of Reiki energy and helps healers act as pure channels for the energy, keeping the healer's personal energy separate. Apophyllite also makes you feel more energetically receptive to Reiki energy, inducing deep relaxation and trust in the process.

TRANSFORMATIONAL POWER

If you have been afraid to look into the deeper causes of your behavior and motivation, meditating with Apophyllite brings the truth gently to the surface so that imbalances can be rectified and karma transmuted to restore harmony to your soul. You can recharge other crystals with the pyramid form or an Apophyllite cluster.

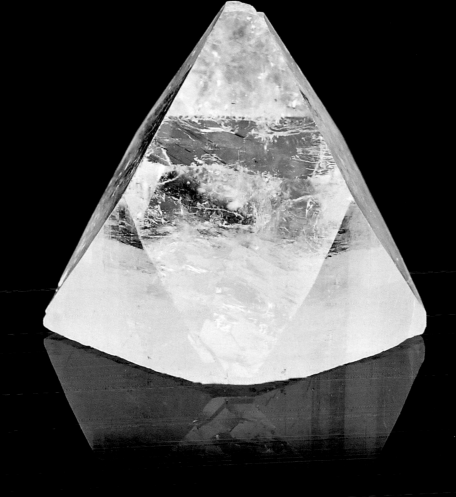

If you are on a spiritual path, meditating with Apophyllite on your third eye promotes inner vision, guidance from the highest level, and total self-awareness.

Aquamarine

- **Chakra correspondences:** Throat, third eye; cleanses and aligns all chakras
- **Physiological correspondences:** Jaw, eyes, liver, throat, thyroid and pituitary glands, hormonal production, growth processes, immune system
- **Vibration:** High

LEGENDARY POWER

Described in antiquity as "a thousand leagues of sunlit sea imprisoned in a cup," Aquamarine's color and strength come from iron. The name means "water of the sea." According to Greek myth, Aquamarine washed ashore after spilling from the jewel casket of the Sirens, legendary seductresses who lured sailors onto the rocks so they could have their way with them. This may be why sailors wore the stone as amulets against sea monsters and to ensure safe voyages. In Roman mythology, Aquamarine was sacred to Neptune, god of the sea.

Aquamarine is a crystal of spiritual vision; it calms your mind, enabling you to reach a high state of awareness. Translucent Aquamarine was used for magic mirrors during the Middle Ages, and seers suspended an Aquamarine ring over a bowl around which the letters of the alphabet were arranged. The ring swung in a manner similar to using a pendulum to spell out answers. Christians at that time believed Aquamarines cleansed their sins.

Gem-quality Aquamarine is found above fourteen thousand feet (4.3 km) on Mount Antero in the Rocky Mountains. Twentieth-century writers Chadbourne and Wright comment that only the hardiest souls venture onto the rugged slopes of this temperamental mountain, known for its tempestuous winds, ice storms, and bitter temperatures—a fitting metaphor for a stone believed to summon the spirits of light to counteract the forces of darkness and assist the soul on its journey to enlightenment.

HEALING POWER

Traditionally, Aquamarine induced calm and healed the eyes, throat, and glands. The Romans used it for stomach, liver, and throat complaints and diseases of the jaw. In *The Vision of Piers Plowman*, Aquamarine miraculously acts as an antidote against poison, reflecting a belief set out in ancient lapidaries. Crystal workers use Aquamarine to harmonize the thyroid and pituitary glands when their functions have been thrown out of balance by psychic overactivity. Place the gem over your throat to free self-expression, over your heart to eliminate fear, and on your brow to sharpen mental perception.

TRANSFORMATIONAL POWER

Aquamarine promotes tolerance and offers support during difficult situations. It helps you overcome judgmental tendencies and take responsibility for yourself. If closure is required, Aquamarine assists in letting go of mental constructs and underlying emotional states. It reminds you that progress is the law of life—the soul must evolve along the pathway it laid down for itself prior to incarnation.

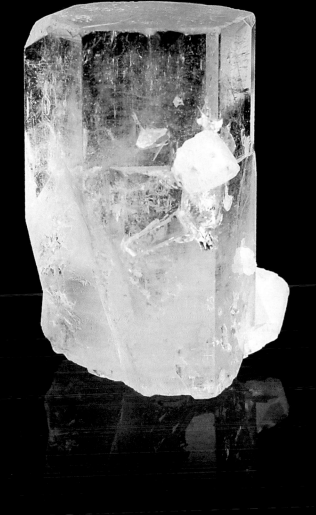

Wear an Aquamarine against
your heart. It inspires hope
in your heart and helps you walk
with enhanced awareness of
your surroundings.

Aragonite

- **Chakra correspondences:** Earth star, base, sacral, soma, throat, third eye, heart, soul star, stellar gateway
- **Physiological correspondences:** Metabolic processes; nervous system; respiratory and immune systems; calcium absorption; disc elasticity; muscles, teeth, bones, lungs, and throat; subtle bodies; polarities
- **Vibration:** Earthy and high

LEGENDARY POWER

Although ancient artifacts from Mexico crafted from Aragonite have been found, their magical and therapeutic properties are lost due to problems with nomenclature. As Aragonite was named after Aragon in Spain, the Alfonso lapidary probably includes this stone, but it is impossible to identify. Aragonite is calcium carbonate, formed from stalactites, and is an excellent Earth healer; it also creates the highest spiritual connection for our planet.

Working with Aragonite reminds us that the Earth is a living, conscious being with whom we must live in synergistic harmony. The stone links you to the Earth's etheric grid and facilitates the planet's own ascension into expanded dimensions, teaching the interconnectedness of all life.

HEALING POWER

An excellent soul healer, Aragonite is also a profoundly physical stone. It is alkaline and warming, especially for the extremities. Positioned over an appropriate spot, anecdotal evidence suggests White Aragonite balances overacidity, reduces joint pain, eases muscle spasms, cramps, and night twitches, and restores circulation to fingers or toes for those with Raynaud's disease. Blue Aragonite assists arthritic conditions and breath work. Use Aragonite-infused water on the scalp to ameliorate hair loss. The stone paradoxically increases energy, yet slows processes that are out of control.

Place Brown Aragonite on the base chakra, Blue on the throat or third eye, and Lilac-pink on the crown to balance the chakras and align them to a flow of higher energies. Brown Aragonite stabilizes the base chakra and grounds the soul comfortably in the physical body.

TRANSFORMATIONAL POWER

Aragonite takes you back into childhood to find the source of angst, anxiety, or dis-ease. The stone's vibrations also convey you to past lives to heal the etheric imprint of karmic wounding or emotional blockages. If you are a hard taskmaster, this patient stone helps you be more forgiving and gentle with yourself, replacing unrealistic expectations with achievable goals. If you suffer from loneliness of the soul, hold delicate Blue Aragonite to call in your spiritual twin flame. (Note: Aragonite is also found in Petrified Wood and Ammolite, mineralized Ammonite).

Beautiful Blue Aragonite contains copper, a mineral considered sacred to Venus. You can put this high-vibration stone on the sacral and base chakras to restore your connection to the divine feminine. Place any of the Aragonites on the earth star chakra to deepen your connection to your spiritual roots in Mother Earth.

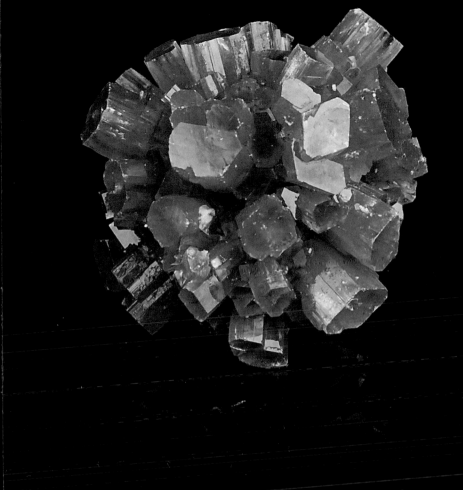

Place Brown Star Aragonite in
the Earth or on a map to facilitate
Earth healing, especially where
geopathic stress has disturbed
the Earth's grid.

Aura Quartzes

- **Chakra correspondences:** All chakras, depending on color; repairs the aura
- **Physiological correspondences:** Thymus, pineal and thyroid glands, immune system, cellular processes, oxygenation of blood, liver, and spleen (effect depends on color and mineral)
- **Vibration:** Aura Quartzes alchemicalized with pure minerals, rather than dyed, reach very high vibrations

LEGENDARY POWER

Aura Quartzes are modern innovations, but rely on the ancient powers of alchemy and synergy to activate their mystical power. Electrostatically bonding precious minerals onto the surface of crystals raises the underlying vibration. Opal, Ruby, and Rose Aura are formed from platinum, Aqua from gold, Sunshine from gold and platinum, Tanzine from gold and indium, Apple from nickel, Flame from titanium and niobium, Tangerine from iron and gold, and Rainbow from titanium and gold. New combinations are constantly being created to generate ever-higher frequencies.

Aura Quartzes activate the lightbody and ground it in the physical body. Laid along the chakras like a rainbow, the various colors raise the vibrational rate of the chakras to accommodate expanded consciousness.

HEALING POWER

The synergistic energy of Aura Quartzes boosts the vibration of the physical body and healing crystal grids, but these stones must be utilized with care. Most Aura Quartzes work at higher vibration levels to accelerate soul evolution through emotional release and karmic healing. Because these synergistic crystals contain a high level of life force, they stimulate the immune and energy systems throughout the body, rapidly detoxifying and increasing the flow of Qi to improve overall well-being.

Tanzine Aura Quartz stimulates the thyroid gland and brings the endocrine system back into alignment, especially when this is blocked by excessive fluoridation. Ruby Aura acts as a subtle antibiotic and eliminates parasites—physical and metaphysical. It transmutes negative emotions such as rage or resentment. Gentler Rose Aura helps you overcome past abuse and infuses the soul with unconditional love, restoring cellular balance. Apple Aura protects the spleen against energy vampires. Dynamic Tangerine Sun penetrates every cell, infusing the body with potent energy to invigorate cellular function and initiate subtle DNA changes. Tangerine Aura also clears third eye blockages.

TRANSFORMATIONAL POWER

Aura Quartzes are a basis for spiritual alchemy and powerful tools for the guidance and expansion of your soul. These crystals deepen your attunement and prepare you for an influx of expanded consciousness. No matter what your underlying problem, there is an Aura Quartz to help you transform negative into positive and recognize the spiritual gifts in your experiences. (Note: Aura Quartzes are brittle, so handle with care. Spurious Aura colors may be dyed rather than alchemicalized, so take care when selecting stones as the dyes may induce an adverse allergic reaction on your skin. See also Anandalite, page 42.)

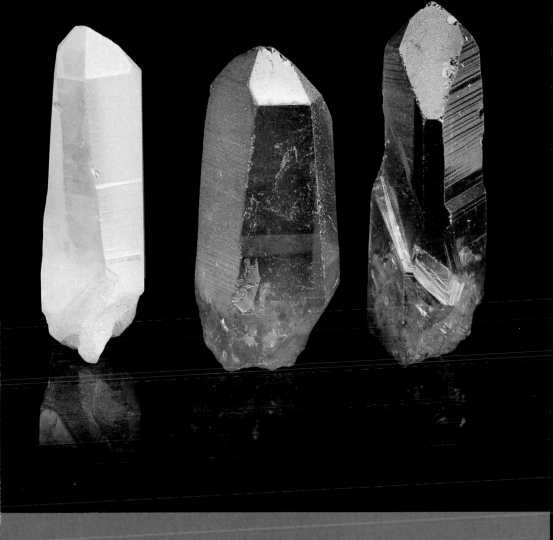

Place Aura Quartz over the heart
seed chakra to release previous
limitations to your spiritual expansion
and free your soul to explore the
multidimensional world.

Aurora Quartz (Anandalite™)

- **Chakra correspondences:** Soul star, stellar gateway, and beyond
- **Physiological correspondences:** Blood cells, fluid systems, central nervous and chakra systems; Anandalite works mainly beyond the physical to activate and harmonize the lightbody into the Earth vibration and to activate subtle neurotransmitters.
- **Vibration:** Exceptionally high

LEGENDARY POWER

Holding Anandalite makes you feel like a lightning conductor for bliss consciousness. Meditating with Anandalite shows us that we have previously operated within a narrow band of awareness, bound by our five senses. Although intuition can transcend the limits of time and space, Anandalite reveals that this can be superseded to move into a quantum field existing everywhere at once, where consciousness is omniscient and omnipresent. It sees all, knows all, and co-creates all.

To know what it feels like to be a particle that is a wave and a wave that is a particle, to travel backward or forward through time, to realize there is no time at all, and that the observer creates the event being observed, meditate with Anandalite. It immerses you in what the ancients called bliss consciousness, divine light, or enlightenment and what today we refer to as Spirit, Source, or Ascension.

You may not be able to explain quantum physics when you emerge, but you will have experienced it. Anandalite introduces a dynamic holographic universe with multidimensional consciousness and mystical interconnectedness. Dissolving the barriers between the different dimensions of creation, it shows the infinite possibilities of the universal mind.

This crystal facilitates kundalini awakening at the highest level, drawing luminescent energy up through the central channel to open the higher crown chakras. It connects you to your higher self with whom a mystical marriage is made, igniting spiritual awakening.

HEALING POWER

Anandalite carries bioscalar waves that activate the body's self-healing mechanism and energetically unclump red and white blood cells. It prepares the central nervous system for a vibrational uplift. To cleanse, purify, and rebalance all chakras, sweep from the base chakra to the higher crown chakras and back again to the earth star to ground the energies. By attuning the energy bodies to a higher frequency, Anandalite anchors the lightbody into the physical.

Anandalite heals dis-ease caused by disharmony between the subtle bodies when they fail to integrate expanded consciousness. If kundalini power is rising in an undirected fashion or expanded consciousness is creating imbalances in the physical body, Anandalite facilitates the integration process. It releases emotional blockages that prevent spiritual awakening.

TRANSFORMATIONAL POWER

This luminescent crystal opens your energy field to divine possibilities and the interconnectedness of all life. It completes the spiritual attunement facilitated by other high-vibration crystals, harmonizing the new frequency so the whole of creation benefits from the quantum uplift.

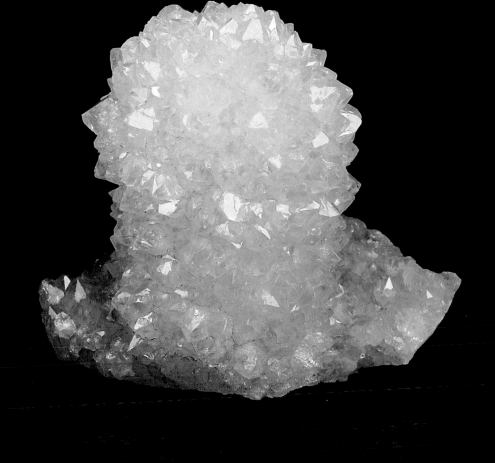

Meditate with Anandalite on your
soma chakra or place it under your
pillow to journey to the highest
spiritual dimensions to awaken
your soul.

Aventurine

- **Chakra correspondences:** Spleen, heart, higher heart (thymus); additional chakras are activated by specific colors
- **Physiological correspondences:** Spleen, eyes, lungs, heart, skin, adrenals, sinuses, muscular and urogenital systems, thymus gland, metabolic processes, nervous system, connective tissue
- **Vibration:** Earthy to high, depending on color

LEGENDARY POWER

A Quartz or Feldspar with Pyrite or Hematite inclusions, Aventurine was known in the ancient world, as numerous statues and amulets attest; however, nomenclature problems make it difficult to assess exactly what properties were attributed to it. *Smargos* was usually translated as Emerald, but could be any green stone, and Aventurine was plentiful in the ancient world whereas Emerald was rare. The "Emerald" in the Breastplate of the High Priest was probably Green Aventurine.

One legend says that an imitation Aventurine, known as Goldstone, was discovered by alchemists as they sought to make gold. Another says that an Italian monastic order made Goldstone according to a secret recipe. The Miotti family made Goldstone in seventeenth-century Venice, and it is now valued as a stone of abundance in its own right.

HEALING POWER

Aventurine is a versatile healing stone. Energetically resonating with the thymus gland and the immune system, it energetically regulates blood pressure and may act as an anti-inflammatory. Its resonance is used to heal arteriosclerosis and decrease cholesterol. Green Aventurine, an all-around healer, works with the heart, adrenals, eyes, and nervous system; it also calms nausea. Blue Aventurine facilitates mental healing, bringing about inner calm. Peach Aventurine enhances the flow of healing energy from the Earth into the physical body. Red Aventurine resonates with the urogenital system to increase fertility and enhance libido. White Aventurine heals the subtle bodies and neurotransmitters.

Crystal workers use Aventurine-infused water to relieve skin conditions. An excellent space and aura protector because it blocks electromagnetic smog, Aventurine is extremely beneficial for sensitive people who respond adversely to emanations from cell phones, Wi-Fi, or computers. This stone also has a powerful connection with the devic kingdom, helping to negate environmental pollution and enhance fertility.

TRANSFORMATIONAL POWER

Aventurine disconnects you from anything that saps your power. It prevents inappropriate relationships from "vampirizating" your heart energy and helps you live within the temple of your own heart.

A stone of joyous abundance, Aventurine assists you in recognizing and overcoming inner feelings of lack that may underlie poverty consciousness. Want to look closely at your future plans, motives, or agendas? Hold Aventurine to focus your mind and see possibilities. If you go outside your comfort zone, this supportive stone increases your confidence, enhances leadership abilities, and helps you step into your true self.

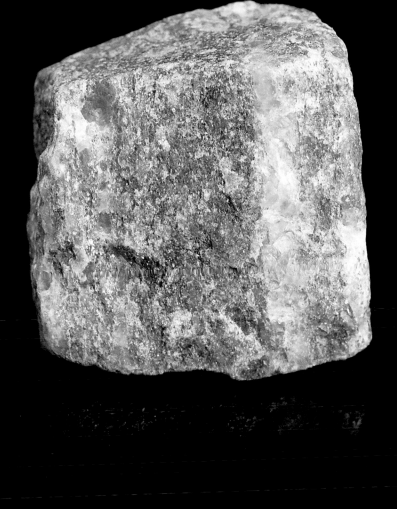

Place Green Aventurine beneath
your left armpit to disconnect
energetic hooks. The stone heals
and seals the site, immediately
raising your energy.

Azeztulite™

- **Chakra correspondences:** Third eye, crown, soul star, stellar gateway, and beyond; connects all chakras to higher dimensions
- **Physiological correspondences:** Cells and cellular processes; works mainly at the spiritual level to facilitate a vibrational shift
- **Vibration:** Exceptionally high

LEGENDARY POWER

Azeztulite's powerful, highly refined energetic qualities usher in a New Age. Raised to an exceptionally pure vibration and infused with "nameless light" by a race of beings called the *Azez*, it is a crystal for accelerated enlightenment. The Azez have stated their purpose as giving spiritual assistance to the Earth and creating an expansion of cellular and cosmic consciousness at this time of vibrational shift.

Azeztulite helps you explore alternative realities and multidimensions, facilitating interdimensional journeys and connections to beings in other realms. It activates all the higher chakras and attunes you to the highest frequencies. However, it should only be used when you have completed your inner work, dissolved ingrained patterns and toxic emotions, and prepared yourself for multidimensional expansion. Otherwise, you may experience side effects such as dizziness, disorientation, or violent emotional outbursts until the new energy is fully assimilated. You might need other crystals to support opening your vibrational potential and to prepare your body for the influx of light and ascent to higher awareness.

If you are just beginning high-vibration crystal work, use the opaque form of Azeztulite. Pink and Golden Azeztulite will take experienced crystal workers ever higher. Pink links you to goddess energy and the wise feminine, Golden to the gods and ancient wisdom. Placed over the third eye, Azeztulite facilitates seeing the future that is being created and the changes needed to bring it into being. Azeztulite's heightened energy can raise the vibration of other stones, especially those in the Quartz family.

HEALING POWER

Azeztulite stimulates cellular consciousness. Exciting but controversial research shows that cell membranes in the body trigger or switch off inherited genetic codes in response to emotions or thoughts. This explains why genetic dis-eases affect some family members and not others. Azeztulite, with its ability to infuse light into the cells, facilitates this control mechanism, activating twelve-strand DNA and stimulating neurotransmitters to heal cellular disorders, which may include tumors and inflammation.

Shifting the physical body to a higher vibration is Azeztulite's most powerful work. By activating and linking "expansion points" at the base of the spine, the dantien, and in the center of the brain, Azeztulite integrates the lightbody into the physical to birth expanded consciousness on Earth.

TRANSFORMATIONAL POWER

Atuning to the "nameless light" carried by Azeztulite offers the opportunity for transformation of the whole planet and everyone on it—spiritual enlightenment for all.

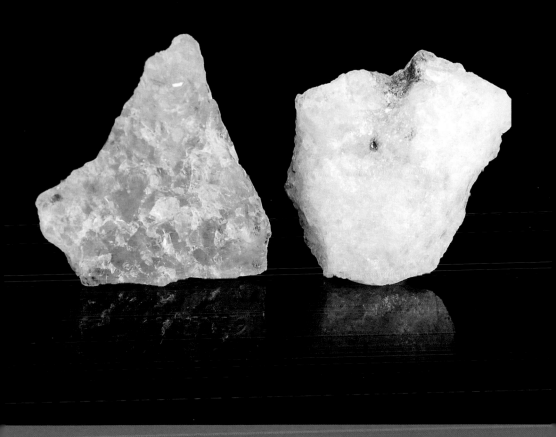

Place Azeztulite on the soul star chakra to create a two-way vibrational ladder between Earth and alternative realities and bring back guidance and spiritual insight.

Banded Agate

- **Chakra correspondences:** Soma, third eye, solar plexus; stabilizes the aura
- **Physiological correspondences:** Eyes; skin; detoxification; oxygen assimilation; cellular function; the brain and cognitive processes; circulatory, urogenital, and nervous systems
- **Vibration:** Earthy

LEGENDARY POWER

Some of the most ancient artifacts were created from Banded Agate, including a five thousand-year-old Mesopotamian amulet inlaid with minute golden writing that called on the power of the planetary god Marduk (Jupiter) to protect the wearer from evil. An even older votive offering, a ceremonial ax carved from Banded Agate, was dedicated to the fearsome weather god, Adad, who threw thunderbolts and lightning. The Egyptians used Banded Agate for amulets to protect their heads. Almost certainly one of the stones in the Breastplate of the High Priest, it perhaps symbolized the All Seeing Eye of God.

Many Banded Agates resemble an eye; therefore, they were considered especially efficacious against the evil eye. They were an indispensable part of a magician's equipment, as the bands controlled the power of the dark spirits being invoked. Banded Agate was also believed to convey the power of sight to statues. A third-century Greek lapidary advises seafarers to wear Banded Agate to safeguard them on the surging ocean.

An eleventh-century description of the eight magical virtues of Agate suggests Banded Agate's power of release. Several virtues involved protection, one in particular against what today would be called "entity possession" or "undue influence," described in those days as "a loathsome fiend" that had secretly attached. According to the lapidary, drinking Agate-infused water immediately detected and removed the astral hitchhiker.

HEALING POWER

A powerful holistic healer, Banded Agate harmonizes the subtle bodies with the physical and removes inner conflict. Placed on appropriate chakras, it enhances cellular memory, assists detoxification, and increases oxygenation in the cells. Botswana Agate supports anyone who wishes to give up tobacco. Gridded around a room, Banded Agate provides healing for the environment and protection against incursion by wandering spirits.

TRANSFORMATIONAL POWER

Agate's bands are a useful vibrational ladder for carrying out subtle healing and past-life soulwork, particularly if, in a previous religious incarnation, the body was regarded as sinful. Pink Botswana Agate gently releases and heals childhood abuse. People who need to learn to love and value themselves can do so under its tender influence. Banded Agate gently reestablishes the notion that sexuality is a normal and natural part of physical incarnation. This stone is especially helpful for children or adults who were sworn to secrecy or who were part of a cult, setting them free to step into their own power. (See Agate, page 20.)

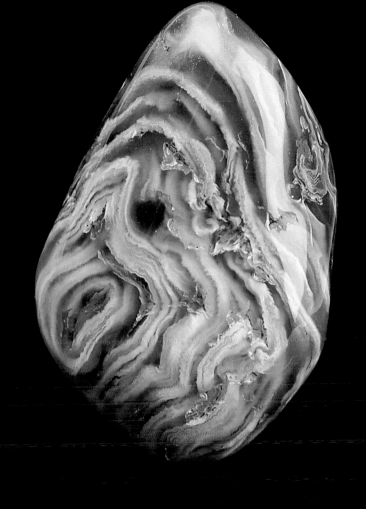

Place Banded Agate on your third
eye to remove ties to any authority
figure who has disempowered you
or whom you have outgrown.

Beryl

- **Chakra correspondences:** Solar plexus, crown, heart; varies according to color and type
- **Physiological correspondences:** Liver, heart, stomach, spine, throat, pulmonary and circulatory systems, detoxification on physical and emotional levels; Golden Beryl (Heliodor): lymphatic system
- **Vibration:** Earthy and high

LEGENDARY POWER

Pliny tells us that ancient Indian craftsmen faceted Beryl into elongated hexagons that enhanced its color, sea green being the most prized (see Aquamarine, page 36). They strung the gem on elephant's bristles. Long before Pliny's time, a spirit was believed to inhabit the stone who, when summoned, revealed secrets. Beryl was also used in rain magic and afforded protection against the storm gods' wrath.

In the Middle Ages Beryl was a popular oracular crystal. Queen Elizabeth I's astrologer and seer, Dr. John Dee, used a polished Beryl ball for scrying. Today Beryl still has the power to stimulate the third eye. The sixteenth-century writer Reginald Scot reported that on praying to St. Helen, "The finest beryl would manifest an image of the saint in an angelic form, and answer any questions asked of her."

Beryl symbolizes happiness and everlasting youth. It had a long association with remembrance of the dead, but opinions varied on exactly how this manifested. The twelfth-century magician Albertus Magnus reported that Beryl had a "horror of death" saying that, although it was particularly potent against evil spirits and demons, the crystal lost its power if it touched a corpse. Nevertheless, Beryl was popular for necromancy, magically calling up the spirits of the dead.

In 1886, S. M. Burnham reported that Beryls several feet in length were occasionally found in Stoneham, Maine. According to him, superior-quality blue Beryls were obtained from the Mourne Mountains in Ireland, but the best stones came from Russia. Beryl is a stone of Archangels Auriel and Zadkiel. It rules the Angelic Dominions.

HEALING POWER

Ancient authorities tell us Beryl healed eye problems. The crystal was rubbed on swollen throats to heal quinsy and placed over the liver to take away pain. Beryl-infused water allegedly cured hiccups. Modern-day crystal workers also use Beryl-infused water as a gargle to soothe throat infections. An antistress remedy, the crystal is applied over the liver and lymphatic system to encourage detoxification. It energetically strengthens the heart, lungs, and circulation.

TRANSFORMATIONAL POWER

An excellent crystal for beginners, gentle Beryl lets you clarify your thoughts and release deeply ingrained beliefs that no longer serve you. Beryl transmutes toxic emotions, leaving only purity of being. The perfect stone for "spiritual constipation," it gets you moving on your soul's path. Its vibration raises your self-esteem and transforms your life.

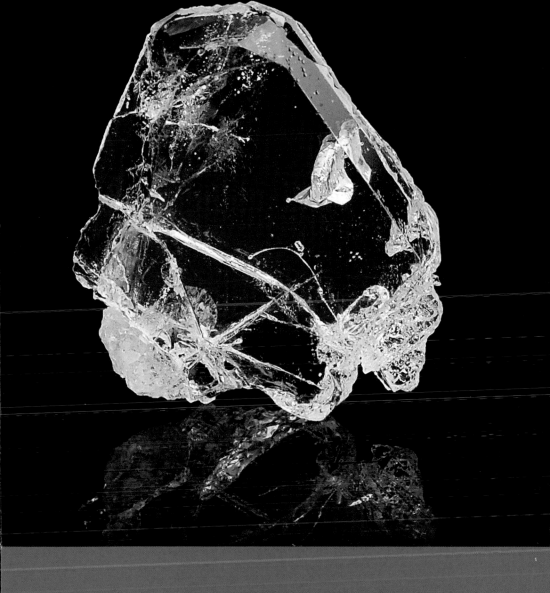

Whenever you feel down, hold
Beryl and remember when you
were totally happy and upbeat.
The memory will remain and see
you through dark times.

Black Tourmaline (Schorl)

- **Chakra correspondences:** Earth star, base, higher heart (thymus); protects all chakras and seals the aura
- **Physiological correspondences:** Immune system, spinal column, detoxification processes, motor function, lungs
- **Vibration:** Earthy

LEGENDARY POWER

Tourmaline is found in many colors due to a variety of chemical constituents, and ancient legends abound about its effectiveness as a protection amulet. Not all ancient sources can be authenticated, however, due to confusion over the name *Schorl*, which is now applied only to Black Tourmaline.

Most Black Tourmaline contains iron, making it a powerfully protective stone. Due to its inner structure, however, Tourmaline traps negative energy within it rather than bouncing it back and forth as iron-based stones are prone to do. Use it in a grid around your home to create a protective shield that blocks negativity or toxic energy of any kind.

Tourmaline is piezoelectric and pyroelectric, generating electricity through pressure or heat, such as from the sun. Due to its attraction-repulsion electrostatic property, it was named the "ash drawer." This property was accidentally discovered by Dutch children, who were playing with the stone. Soon afterward, Dutch mariners began using the stone to draw ash out of their long-stemmed pipes. The Chinese used Burmese Black Tourmalines to make buttons for Mandarins' hats.

HEALING POWER

Black Tourmaline protects the body against electromagnetic stress, negativity, and psychic attack. It may help to harmonize the brain and repattern neural pathways in malfunctions, such as dyslexia or dyspraxia. Realigning the spinal column, Black Tourmaline energetically stimulates the immune system and the thyroid gland. To relieve pain and arthritic swelling, hold this stone over the site.

TRANSFORMATIONAL POWER

Black Tourmaline is invaluable for sensitive people who are overwhelmed by geopathic or electromagnetic stress, including Wi-Fi, or by radiation. It draws the toxicity out through your feet and transmutes it into powerful Earth-healing energy. Wear Black Tourmaline at your throat or place it on your computer or other electrical equipment to block emanations and strengthen your auric field.

Wearing Black Tourmaline gives psychic protection, too. To transmute negative energy, place the stone on the name of the person who is instigating an attack.

At a psychological level, Black Tourmaline helps you understand how holding onto toxic emotions or negative thoughts attacks you from within, creating dis-ease that ultimately manifests physically. The stone supports you in acting and thinking positively, so you create a beneficial environment for yourself.

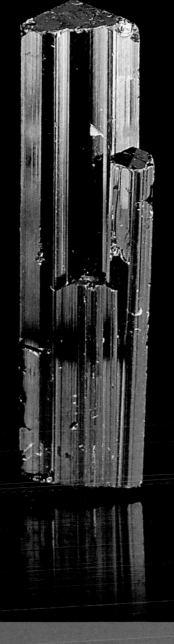

To instantly stop jealousy,
ill will, or all-out psychic attack,
wear Black Tourmaline over
your thymus. The stone safely
defuses the attack.

Bloodstone (Heliotrope)

- **Chakra correspondences:** Base, sacral, higher heart (thymus); cleanses and realigns the lower chakras

- **Physiological correspondences:** Blood and circulation, kidneys, adrenals, liver, gallbladder, spleen, bladder, intestines, metabolic processes, detoxification, acidification balance, immune and lymphatic systems

- **Vibration:** Earthy

LEGENDARY POWER

Bloodstone has long been famed for its magical power in controlling the weather and banishing evil. Throughout the ancient and medieval world, Bloodstone was worn as an amulet. One of the earliest known healing stones, Bloodstone occurs in a five-thousand-year-old Mesopotamian "recipe" for purifying the blood—which negates later legends that the stone was formed at the crucifixion when Christ's blood fell onto Jasper at the foot of the cross. Bloodstone was said to have the power of healing wounds. Its coagulant effect probably comes from the iron oxide in the stone.

Pliny noted the stone was believed to confer invisibility on the wearer, a possibility he repudiated, however.

In the language of gemstones, Bloodstone signifies courage and wisdom. According to the magician Agrippa, it ensured fame and long life. The Victorians wore it to signal "I mourn your absence." Heliotrope and Bloodstone are often conflated, especially in early lapidaries, but Heliotrope is translucent whereas Bloodstone is opaque.

HEALING POWER

In the Middle Ages, Bloodstone was credited with the power to stop nosebleeds, but its connection with blood and the kidneys dates back to Mesopotamia. In the ancient Near East and in Europe in the Middle Ages, it was powdered and mixed with honey and egg white to draw out snake venom, reduce tumors, and staunch hemorrhages.

According to the Alfonso lapidary, Bloodstone hung over an abscess cleared putrefaction in a day—and just looking at a Bloodstone apparently prevented eye diseases. The powder traditionally dried watery secretions because of the stone's great heat and dryness. Today crystal workers use Bloodstone to strengthen the blood and kidneys, and to cleanse subtle energy. It is still said to reduce the formation of pus and to prevent overacidification.

TRANSFORMATIONAL POWER

Bloodstone protects the soul on many levels, keeping out undesirable entities and dispelling mental confusion. Regarded as a shape-shifting stone because its colors change in different lights, it teaches you how to travel invisibly between the worlds and negotiate different realms. In everyday life, Bloodstone shows when it is appropriate to strategically withdraw from situations, but instills the courage to confront threats when necessary. Carry it if you need to adjust to new circumstances. This stone heals the ancestral line (see Glossary on page 216) by dispelling negative patterns, helping you live in the present untrammeled by the past. With Bloodstone raising your vibrations, you become a purified being.

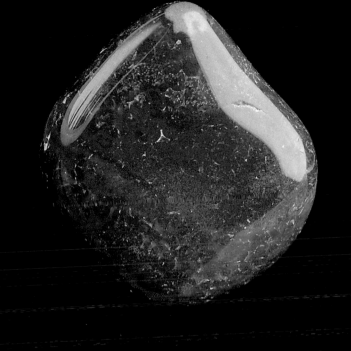

Place Bloodstone over the thymus (higher heart chakra) to stimulate your immune system and ward off colds and influenza.

Blue Lace Agate

- **Chakra correspondences:** Throat, third eye, crown, heart
- **Physiological correspondences:** Eyes, throat, shoulders, neck, thyroid gland, stomach, uterus, lymphatic and digestive systems, skeletal system, pancreas, capillaries
- **Vibration:** Earthy

LEGENDARY POWER

Blue Lace Agate is a comparatively recent find, but Blue Agates have been prized as communication enhancers since ancient times. According to the fourth-century Greco-Roman Orphic *Lithica*, Blue Agate conveys to the wearer grace and persuasive power of speech:

> *Adorned with this, thou woman's heart shall gain*
> *And by persuasion thy desire obtain;*
> *And if of men thou aught demand, shalt come*
> *With all thy wishes fulfilled rejoicing home.*

The eleventh-century Marbod lapidary confirms, "the wearer of an agate shall be made agreeable and persuasive to man, and have the favour of God." A couple of centuries later Bernard Mandeville said, "it makes one a beautiful speaker and gracious with words . . . and helps one to acquire intelligence and sense." And in 1585, Gerolamo Cardano insisted that an Agate helped him succeed in negotiations and win debates, saying it made him "temperate, continent, and cautious."

According to modern crystal lore, Blue Lace Agate instills the ability to analyze and dissect, and focuses the mind. Placed on the third eye, this stone opens the inner eye to help you intuitively see beyond the confines of consensual reality.

HEALING POWER

Modern crystal workers use gentle Blue Lace Agate to instill peace of mind. It opens the throat chakra to encourage free expression of thoughts and feelings that previously have been blocked. Blocked feelings are one of the most common sources of dis-ease, and the stone gently dissolves this repression. Such blockages may be reflected in psychosomatic shoulder or throat problems, which can be released by placing Blue Lace Agate on the throat chakra. Positioned on the throat, its vibrations restore energetic balance to the thyroid and parathyroid glands, assisting metabolic function.

Water infused with Blue Lace Agate makes an excellent gargle for sore throats and has been used to regulate the fluid balance in the brain.

TRANSFORMATIONAL POWER

Blue Lace Agate dramatically changes your ability to communicate and to speak your truth. It is especially beneficial for healing psychosomatic ailments that arise from not being able to express your feelings, or from having been sworn to secrecy in this or a previous lifetime. In situations where you fear you will be judged or ridiculed, the stone can be extremely helpful. It also ameliorates feelings of anger that may have arisen in the past and promotes forgiveness. (See also Agate on page 20 and Banded Agate on page 40.)

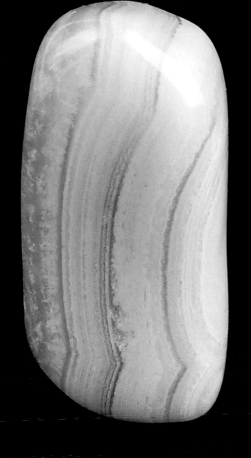

Wear Blue Lace Agate at your
throat to voice your most
profound personal and spiritual
truths, or to heal a sore throat.

Blue Moonstone

- **Chakra correspondences:** Soma, third eye, crown, soul star, stellar gateway, higher heart (thymus), heart seed
- **Physiological correspondences:** Female reproductive system, lymphatic system, metabolic processes, digestive tract, pineal gland, skin, hair, eyes, hyperactivity, biorhythms, subtle energy bodies
- **Vibration:** White Moonstone low, Rainbow Moonstone high, natural Blue Moonstone extremely high

LEGENDARY POWER

Blue Moonstone occurs naturally in Sri Lanka and parts of India. The legendary power of Moonstone lies in its connections with the moon, and it traditionally stimulated metaphysical abilities. Dedicated to Diana, Roman goddess of the moon, the crystal bestowed wisdom and victory on the wearer. Pliny tells us Moonstone changed according to the moon's phases, becoming more brilliant at the full moon. Its adularescence—a ghostly shining on the surface—is created by water in the crystal.

In the Middle Ages, Moonstone was a love talisman during the waxing moon—love increased as the moon grew bigger. During the waning period, Moonstone enabled the wearer to see the future. In some cultures, Moonstone was placed under the tongue to activate its properties, linking it to the central channel through which Qi and kundalini energy flow.

Moonstone is a sacred Hindu stone. A spirit that resides in the stone is believed to bring good fortune to its owner. Moonstone is linked with Archangel Gabriel.

HEALING POWER

Moonstone traditionally prevented lunacy and calmed the soul. It regulated menstruation and menopause. Blue Moonstone may help to bring the female reproductive system to optimum energetic functioning prior to conception. Placed over the thymus, Blue Moonstone energetically attunes the physical body to assimilate the minerals and nutrients required for lightbody integration.

TRANSFORMATIONAL POWER

Common white Moonstone can induce delusions, but these are turned into profound spiritual insights by Blue Moonstone, which activates your expanded consciousness and awakens your spiritual potential. If you are new to crystal working, placing the three types of Moonstone successively on the soma chakra facilitates ascension through the vibratory levels. White Moonstone opens your metaphysical abilities and prepares you for an influx of spiritual energy. Rainbow Moonstone infuses you with cosmic and spiritual light, so you are part of an ever-unfolding continuous cycle of life and consciousness. Blue Moonstone takes you to the peak of coherent multidimensional awareness, enabling you to be "here" and "there" simultaneously.

Gentle Blue Moonstone helps a "macho" man get in touch with his inner feminine qualities or an overly aggressive female to find her gentler side. Using this crystal balances the polarities of masculine and feminine and prepares you for alchemical marriage and androgynous *being*. (Note: If Blue Moonstone energy is difficult to assimilate, hold Hematite to reground yourself. You may need to remove Blue Moonstone at full moon.)

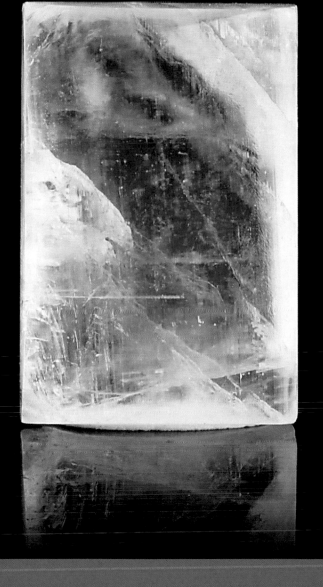

Place a Blue Moonstone on the
back of your neck for ten minutes
to relax muscle tension and
increase blood flow to the brain.

Brandenberg

- **Chakra correspondences:** Activates all chakras including soul star, stellar gateway, and beyond
- **Physiological correspondences:** Etheric blueprint, limbic brain, neurotransmitters; nervous, cellular, electrical, metabolic, and immune systems
- **Vibration:** Exceptionally high

LEGENDARY POWER

Brandenberg has exceptional power and clarity, attuned to pure consciousness. It carries the hologram of your soul. A master healer, it is the most versatile multidimensional healing tool on the planet. If you can only have one crystal, make it a Brandenberg. It does all you ask—and more than you ever dreamed possible. This amazing crystal is found at the crossroads of powerful meridians that feed the soul energy of the Earth's matrix. It is a key to planetary healing and the expansion process.

Containing the energetic resonance of Amethyst, Smoky, and Clear Quartz, Brandenberg works synergistically to restore balance at the physical, emotional, mental, ancestral, planetary, karmic, and spiritual levels. Its phantoms, or bubbles, can be intuitively traversed to explore all the levels of being.

Brandenberg releases entities, thought forms and mental constructs or influences, karmic imprints or connections, and soul imperatives that no longer serve. Holding a Brandenberg takes you into the most perfect energetic state possible. It sets your soul free to fulfill your present-life soul purpose. Meditating with a Brandenberg pinpoints conditions you assumed for the purpose of your soul's growth. It takes you back to forks in the road to reframe choices you previously made, seeding the future with potential. Highlighting the gift in any experience, it moves you forward on your soul path.

HEALING POWER

By taking you back to the perfect blueprint that existed before the soul's journey began, a Brandenberg energetically retunes core vibrational patterns. It aligns all systems of the body to optimum functioning and brings forward a perfection of being that can be reflected in body and soul. A tool for profound cellular healing and twelve-strand DNA activation, it creates new neural pathways as it triggers the cell membrane to remember it is a vehicle of conscious evolution.

With its ability to cut ties and release old soul covenants, this crystal is extremely beneficial for energetic depletion, whether from a past or present life source. Brandenberg is a powerful karmic cleanser that reprograms your brain to a new energetic pattern and resets your immune system response to optimum. Existing at the energetic interface where consciousness becomes matter, Brandenberg acts as a gatekeeper against psychic attack, holding your whole being in positive spiritual light. It facilitates high spiritual guidance.

TRANSFORMATIONAL POWER

Brandenberg helps you realize you are perfect exactly as you are in this present moment.

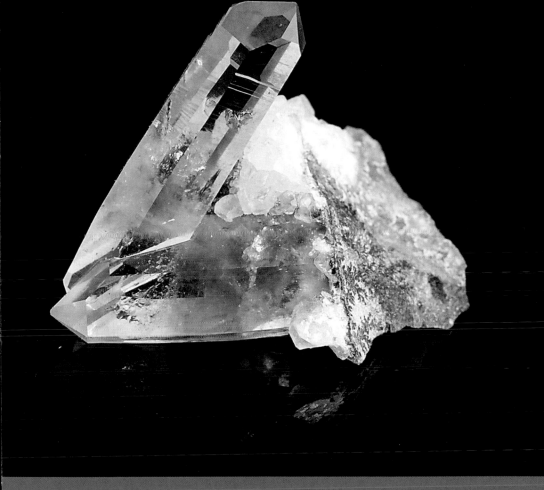

HARNESSING THE POWER

Mentally call your Brandenberg to
you before you set out to find the
physical crystal. There will be one
that is uniquely *yours*.

Bronzite

- **Chakra correspondences:** Earth star, base, sacral; activates and synthesizes all chakras
- **Physiological correspondences:** Blood; cells; biochemical processes, including assimilation of iron and alkaline-acid balance; nervous and circulatory systems
- **Vibration:** Earthy

LEGENDARY POWER

Bronzite's power lies in its iron core. Ancient humans considered iron a gift from the gods because it came from the sky as meteorites. The Roman historian Plutarch referred to it as the "bones of the gods." Having passed through the heat of Earth's atmosphere, meteoric iron did not need smelting and could be worked cold, so it was used millennia before iron was extracted from the Earth. The earliest iron artifacts date back seven thousand years.

Iron is a vital constituent in the human organism, essential for transport of hemoglobin in red blood cells and other cellular structures. Without iron, the body's vitality is low and cannot sustain biochemical processes. Bronzite may aid chronic exhaustion, dramatically improving core strength. It balances masculine and feminine energies within the body or psyche. This stone helps you be more assertive, in standing up for yourself and in decision making.

Sold as a magical protector, Bronzite must be used with care because it may amplify and exacerbate the effects of ill intent, spells, and psychic attack. The energy bounces between attacker and attacked. Adding Black Tourmaline to the crystal mix stops the energetic attack and cuts the connection permanently.

Bronzite energetically cleanses your environment, transmuting negative energies and creating a ring of protection. Within that space, you learn the value of non-doing, experiencing dynamic *being*. This powerful shamanic stone takes you journeying through other worlds to find your power animal, and guides you to the core of your true self.

HEALING POWER

Crystal healers use Bronzite's power to energetically increase the assimilation of iron, boosting the circulation of red blood cells, and to enhance the passage of energy throughout the subtle meridians of the body. A pain reliever, it may regulate overacidity and prevent muscle cramps. Wear or grid it if Wi-Fi emanations are detrimental to your well-being.

TRANSFORMATIONAL POWER

Bronzite's strong magnetic flow provides an inner compass to assist in finding your direction: physically and spiritually. If you tend to judge other people or yourself harshly, Bronzite teaches the power of compassion and forgiveness. If you feel powerless in a situation or have handed your power over to someone else, holding Bronzite calls your power back and helps you take the course of right action. Conversely, if you have been overly willful, especially in past lives, Bronzite teaches you to attune your will so you are guided by your soul rather than your ego.

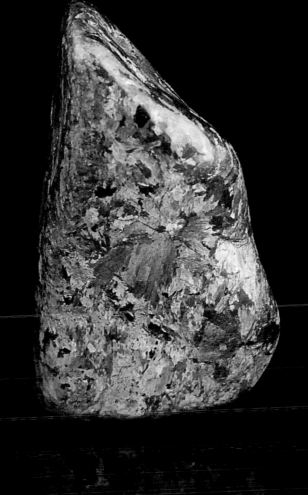

To create a safe, sacred space
for meditation, lay out tumbled
Bronzites to form a six-pointed
star with a stone at each point.

Carnelian

- **Chakra correspondences:** Base, sacral
- **Physiological correspondences:** Blood and blood-rich organs, metabolic processes, reproductive organs, mineral assimilation
- **Vibration:** Earthy

LEGENDARY POWER

An ancient rhyme states, "Fate has with virtues great Carnelian's nature graced; tied round the neck or on the finger placed." A popular stone for seals and amulets throughout the Mediterranean and Near East, Carnelian was common in ancient times. As Pliny points out, it prevented misfortune and attracted good luck. It appears in an early Mesopotamian recipe for fighting off disease and, with Jasper, was tied around the wrists of Egyptian newborns. A seventeenth-century English lapidary says it "recreates the minde, cohabits sad dreams, expels fear, and preserves the carrier from witches and harms." Goethe tells us, "It brings good luck to child and man [and] drives away all evil things. To thee and thine protection brings." In the Arabic world, the name of Allah engraved on a Carnelian protected the wearer from harm, and legend says the Prophet Mohammed wore one mounted in silver.

The Alfonso lapidary says, "men love this stone because of its beauty and its virtues." Virtues included helping people involved in court cases; if an advocate speaking on their behalf wore Carnelian, it helped him argue eloquently and fearlessly. Carnelian also attracted whatever you most desired. In modern crystal working, it is a popular stone for abundance rituals.

HEALING POWER

The Alfonso lapidary suggests wearing Carnelian if you have a weak voice, as it energizes the throat. The stone staunched bleeding, especially in women whose menstrual flow was great, and it was pulverized for use as toothpaste, a cavity and gum healer. Modern crystal workers prize Carnelian for its ability to energize. It may benefit infertility, impotence, and frigidity. By the system of "like heals like," its energetic signature calms inflammation, increases mineral assimilation, and lifts depression.

TRANSFORMATIONAL POWER

Carnelian stimulates courage and action. It restores motivation, energizes the soul body, and helps turn dreams into realities. With this stone, you can work an act of truly outrageous magic that transmogrifies the mundane world. For instance, use it to successfully apply for a dream job, for which you are not qualified, where you dramatically transform other people's lives.

Traditionally, Carnelian protected against envy. Eastern belief said that if you envied anyone's possessions or wealth, your thoughts caused him to lose what you craved. This is useful karmic insight into the power of envy. Magnanimous Carnelian helps you be grateful for what you have and to give thanks for the good fortune of others, reinforcing universal abundance.

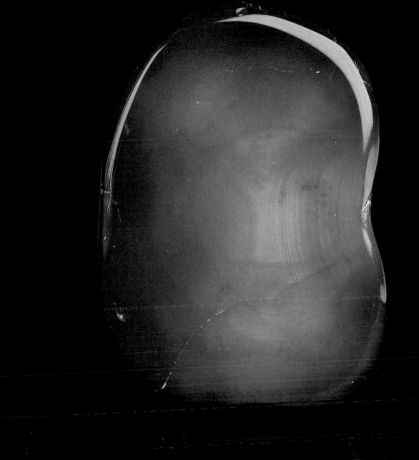

Place a Carnelian where you
will see it often. Each time
you pass the stone, touch it
and say, "I am grateful."

Cathedral Quartz

- **Chakra correspondences:** Past life, soma, crown, soul star, stellar gateway, and beyond
- **Physiological correspondences:** Pain relief, multidimensional cellular processes, viruses
- **Vibration:** Very high

LEGENDARY POWER

This Library of Light holds all possibilities and knowledge of past, present, and future; it is attuned to the Akashic Record. This Quartz formation has emerged now to assist in shifting the vibrational frequency of our planet and all who live here. I use one to help download information from the crystal oversouls regarding the deeper purposes of new crystals.

Cathedral Quartz has many terminations coming off its main body, symbolizing the oneness of creation. It reminds us that, although we may experience ourselves as individuals, at the core level we are all one. In group work, Cathedral Quartz harmonizes and amplifies group intention, acting as both receiver and transmitter for group energy.

HEALING POWER

Cathedral Quartz has the master healing power of Quartz taken to a higher dimension, to work on cellular memory from the vibration of light. This crystal heals dis-eases carried through the ancestral line or by your own soul. Physically, anecdotal evidence suggests it is magical for relieving pain and for preventing bacterial and viral infections. (Place it directly over the affected site.)

TRANSFORMATIONAL POWER

Cathedral Quartz lets you access the fullness of your whole being and the history of your soul. It helps you remember who you truly are and why you assumed incarnation. Through working with Cathedral Quartz, you develop an unshakeable sense of your true value and reason for being. Each type of Cathedral Quartz has its own specific transformation power.

Clear Cathedral Quartz sheds light on every part of your being, purifying and activating your core perfection as a child of the universe. Citrine Cathedral Quartz is excellent for releasing poverty consciousness. It takes you back to your roots to examine your core beliefs about prosperity, helps you recognize your inner riches, and reprograms your soul to always expect enough. By reminding you of the power of personal intention and the abundant universe, it enhances awareness of your own worth and attracts abundance to you. Smoky Cathedral Quartz transmutes negativity at any level. This is a powerful crystal for soul healing and karmic transformation. The smallest piece is potent, especially when used in grids. Invaluable if negative thoughts and toxic emotional patterns are causing dis-ease, this crystal brings in light and elevates vibrations to a place where negativity cannot take hold.

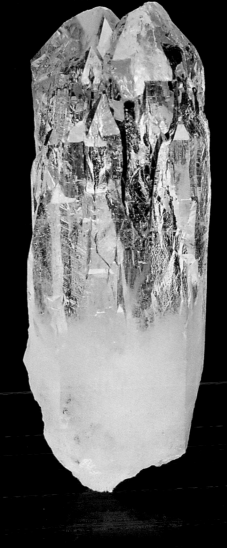

Meditate with Cathedral Quartz
daily to raise the frequency of
your mind, encouraging positive
thought and intention.

Celestite

- **Chakra correspondences:** Throat, third eye, crown, soul star, stellar gateway
- **Physiological correspondences:** Eyes, ears, throat, muscles, cellular structures
- **Vibration:** High

LEGENDARY POWER

Named from the Latin *caelestis*—literally "celestial" or "heavenly"—Celestite in its ethereal blue form is a potent crystal for cosmic connection. Gazing on it lifts you to another dimension and instills a profound sense of peace as it expands your consciousness and promotes harmonious coexistence with the whole cosmos. This crystal offers a ray of hope similar to seeing the sun in the depths of winter. It assures you there is light in the darkness and that warmth will return.

The heavenly blue of Celestite may be created by minute traces of gold or natural irradiation in the crystal, reminding us of the golden spark of pure spirit in our hearts. Its potency, however, comes from the mineral strontium, which paradoxically is used in making red fireworks—there is a powerful force at the heart of this delicate-looking crystal.

Modern crystal lore says an angelic choir created Celestite, and one of the stone's major properties is angelic communication. Keep this crystal with you at all times to call in your guardian angel. Blue Celestite is associated with Archangel Michael, and Lilac Celestite (Lilac Anhydrite) is a stone of Zadkiel.

HEALING POWER

This gentle crystal energetically infuses cell memory with a higher vibration, switching on positive genetic potential and dissolving dis-ease carried in the genes or in cellular memory to restore order within the cell. Crystal workers place it on the body to relax muscle tension and heal throat conditions.

TRANSFORMATIONAL POWER

Meditating with Celestite connects you to the celestial wisdom of the universal mind and creates a sanctuary for your soul. If you are new to crystal power, Celestite is the perfect crystal to bring you into contact with other dimensions. Its gentle, opening effect creates a peaceful space in which to safely explore your inner being and/or your higher self.

If you are beset by fears and worries, meditating with Celestite clears confusion, inducing hope and mental clarity. By helping you to come from your heart rather than your head, this crystal synthesizes instinct and intuition. It is the perfect crystal for artists who need to stimulate creativity and expand their ideas.

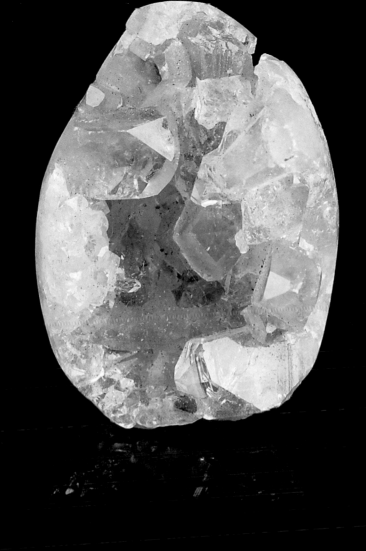

Place Celestite on your third eye
to open psychic communication
with angelic realms and connect to
the star beings of the Pleiades.

Chlorite Quartz

- **Chakra correspondences:** Heart, higher heart (thymus), earth star; cleanses all chakras
- **Physiological correspondences:** Immune system, detoxification, assimilation of minerals and vitamins
- **Vibration:** Earthy to high

LEGENDARY POWER

Chlorite has incredible cleansing abilities, especially when its properties are synergistically amplified by Quartz. Chlorite's complex internal structure traps and transmutes negative energy, purifying your personal energy field, and realigning the spiritual and physical bodies and the environment in which they exist.

Chlorite appears in a Quartz point as a solid form or ghostlike phantom. Phantom crystals hold the memory of all that has been. This formation puts the past into perspective, breaking old patterns so that new growth can occur. Because phantoms were laid down in layers, they help you see how the "layers" of your soul developed during physical incarnations. Chlorite points also assist in removing energetic implants, cleansing the physical or subtle bodies, and restoring energetic function.

Chlorite resonates with Raphael, the Archangel of healing and purification, and is an effective environmental purifier. Chlorite points create a sacred space for meditation or healing work—aim their points away from your space to draw off negative energies. Keep a large Chlorite in a therapy room to transmute negative energies released during healing work.

HEALING POWER

Chlorite clears built-up stagnant energy from the body and energetically removes toxins at every level. As Chlorite may encourage the proliferation of helpful bacteria, it can be placed on the abdomen following a course of antibiotic treatment to stimulate beneficial bacteria to repopulate the gut. Bathing with Chlorite-infused water may remove age spots and growths.

A useful antidote to anxiety and panic attacks, Chlorite Quartz can be worn to energetically stabilize bipolar disorder and other psychiatric conditions (under the guidance of an experienced crystal therapist).

TRANSFORMATIONAL POWER

If you have had images, visual templates, or other symbols inserted into your energy field or your mind—especially ones that were deliberately intertwined with your brain cells—and these have not proved to be for your highest good, Chlorite Quartz gently sucks them out. The crystal's Quartz light infuses the space without damaging the neural field, reprogramming cellular memory to assist your highest potential. If a lost spirit has attached itself to the auric field, a Chlorite point helps the entity detach and move to the light, so that it completes its transition.

Chlorite releases frustration, jealousy, and resentment from the heart. By radiating compassion and forgiveness, it helps you value everyone's uniqueness. This crystal promotes self-realization in a grounded way, showing your soul's breadth and its place on the Earth plane.

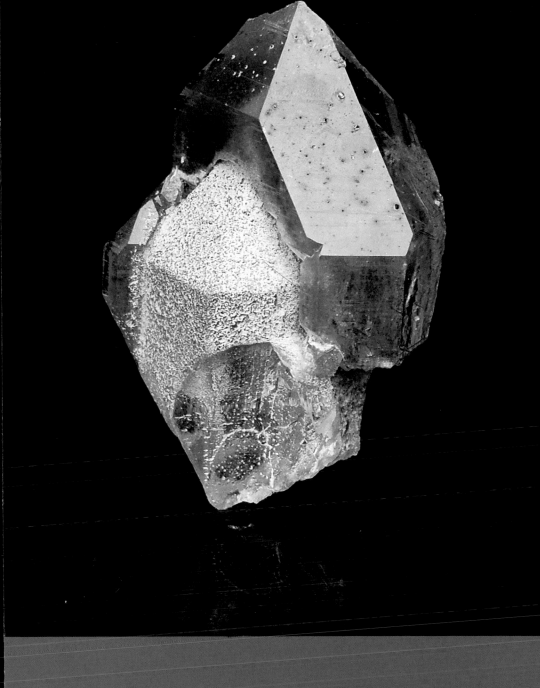

Place a Chlorite point down in the
tank of your toilet to continuously
flush away negative energies and
keep your home energetically pure.

Chrysocolla

- **Chakra correspondences:** Sacral; cleanses and activates all chakras, uniting you with the divine
- **Physiological correspondences:** Pancreas, blood and circulation, brain, bones, muscles, thyroid gland, throat, and digestive, reproductive, and metabolic systems
- **Vibration:** Earthy to high, depending on type

LEGENDARY POWER

Many early stone names were generic, and when writers such as Theophrastus and Pliny mention *chrysokolla* they could be referring to Malachite (see page 122) or Chrysocolla. The name means "gold glue" due to its ancient use in intricate gold work. *The Leyden Papyrus*, an Egyptian scientific and medicinal text, includes a recipe for gold solder. The chrysokolla base was heated with a reducing agent to produce copper, which bonded to the gold *in situ*. Whether the base stone was Malachite or Chrysocolla is unclear as both were found in Egyptian copper mines. The Alfonso lapidary also refers to a "joiner of gold" that cleaved everything together no matter how small the amount. The joiner of gold also cleaned out ulcers, healed scabies of the eyes, and reattached retinas—all properties traditionally associated with Chrysocolla.

Whether we are referring to the extraction of copper or the joining of gold, this is an allegory for the transmutation of the soul through spiritual alchemy. The process resonates with Chrysocolla as the stone transmutes negative energy of all kinds, reconnecting you to the divine within.

HEALING POWER

Traditionally Chrysocolla is used as a powerful detoxifier and relaxant that relieves cramps and ensures peaceful sleep. Placed under the pillow, it prevented nightmares. This stone was said to stimulate metabolism and assist the eyes and throat. It reduced infection, goiter, and inflammations such as gout. Combined with Smoky Quartz, it may facilitate clearing fungal infections. Crystal workers use it to stimulate liver function and energetically mobilized heavy metals out of the body. A powerful energizer for body and psyche, it transforms lethargy at any level.

Drusy Chrysocolla calms physical or emotional trauma. Placed on the lower chakras, Crystalline Chrysocolla (Gem Silica) may help to heal sexual trauma from the current or a past life, particularly if this has involved magical or cult ritual.

TRANSFORMATIONAL POWER

Tranquil Chrysocolla assists you in moving away from egocentricity, aligning your behavior with personal ideals. Worn at the throat, it helps you live in accordance with your truth and speak your beliefs calmly and fluently. It eases judgment and encourages compassion and forgiveness for those who oppose you. If you are dependent on others, the stone instills a sense of trust in yourself, encouraging independence as it gently supports the soul. Crystalline Chrysocolla has a higher vibration than the base stone and increases the rate at which energies are raised and stabilized.

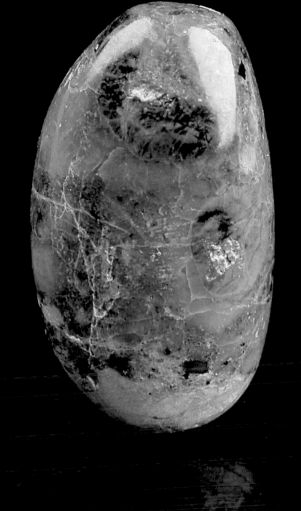

Place Chrysocolla in warm
bathwater to infuse your whole
being with peace and tranquility.

Cinnabar

- **Chakra correspondences:** Base and sacral
- **Physiological correspondences:** Blood, reproductive system
- **Vibration:** Earthy

LEGENDARY POWER

In ancient Egypt, alchemy was not a search for gold, the philosopher's stone, or an elixir of eternal life (the quest that drove medieval and Chinese alchemy), but a process by which the power of the gods was circulated and creation maintained. Alchemy symbolized a soul dying to the material world and being reborn again in spiritual splendor: a process in which the microcosm, the soul, reflected the glory of the macrocosm, the cosmos.

The Egyptian alchemist Cleopatra stated, "the highest descends to the lowest, and the lowest rises to the highest," paraphrasing the aphorism from the Emerald Tablet of Hermes Trismegistus.

It doth ascend from earth to heaven; again it doth descend to earth and unites in itself the forces from things superior and things inferior . . . This thing is the strongest of all powers, the force of all forces, for it overcometh every subtle thing and doth penetrate every solid substance. Thus was the world created.

To the ancients, Cinnabar magically produced "quicksilver" (mercury) from within itself. In the first century B.C.E., Vitruvius tells us that Cinnabar, when struck with a hammer, shed tears of quicksilver. Extraction of mercury was also an alchemical process. Out of the red stone came shining metal that magically separated and recombined itself.

The Leyden Papyrus gives a recipe for using Cinnabar to prepare gold ink to control the gods, and Cinnabar's use in Stone Age cave paintings may have a magical basis. The ancient Persians called Cinnabar dragon's blood because of its fiery nature. In the East, Cinnabar was traditionally kept in cash boxes to attract abundance. Cinnabar is a stone for Archangel Michael.

HEALING POWER

Despite Cinnabar's toxicity, Chinese medicine has used the stone for over five thousand years. It enhanced fertility. In the Middle Ages, mercury treated venereal diseases, although the cure was more dangerous than the disease. Crystal workers today use Cinnabar to purify the blood and increase strength and vigor.

TRANSFORMATIONAL POWER

Cinnabar facilitates physical, emotional, mental, and spiritual alchemy, and reminds you that the body is a crucible for the soul. Heightening assertiveness without inducing aggression, it releases energy blockages and realigns the chakras. It lets you recognize the divinity of all things and see that higher dimensions interpenetrate lower. Cinnabar enables the soul to raise its vibrations to the highest frequency, harnessing the power of the gods. (Note: Wash hands thoroughly after use.)

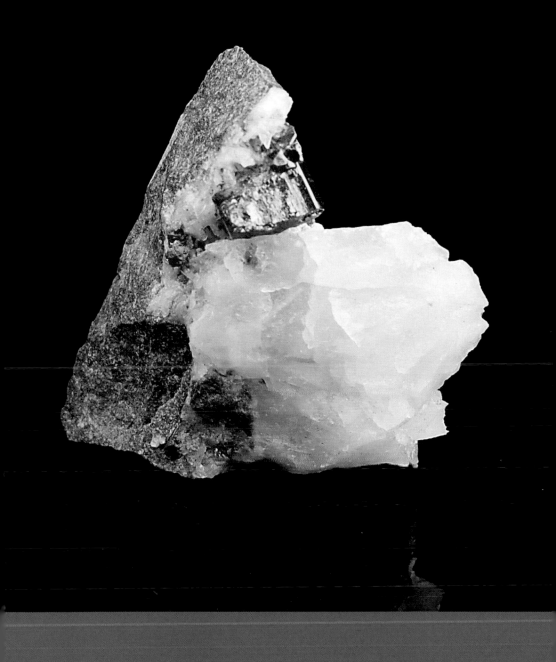

Place tumbled Cinnabar stones
on your base and crown chakras
to activate your central energy
channel and stimulate spiritual
alchemy at your core.

Citrine

- **Chakra correspondences:** Sacral; cleanses and energizes all chakras
- **Physiological correspondences:** Detoxification, circulation and energy systems, thymus and thyroid glands, spleen, pancreas, kidneys, bladder, female reproductive system
- **Vibration:** High

LEGENDARY POWER

Long known as the Merchant Stone, Citrine is associated with abundance and prosperity consciousness. Drawing abundance to you requires mental and emotional focus combined with the power of intention. Much more than mere wealth and possessions, prosperity is a state of mind that recognizes your own inner riches and trusts the universe to provide appropriately for your needs.

Using Citrine raises your self-esteem, gives you confidence, and helps you to value yourself for who you are rather than what you do or own. It lets you live in the moment rather than dreaming of what might be. Citrine gives you energy to manifest your own reality and to attract everything you need.

HEALING POWER

Citrine invigorates the body and activates the immune system. Beneficial for degenerative dis-eases, it encourages energy flow and balances hormones. Citrine energy enriches the spleen and pancreas, and combats infections or pain in the urogenital tract. Citrine-infused water is traditionally used to alleviate menstrual cramps and chronic fatigue.

TRANSFORMATIONAL POWER

Abundance is about living fully on all levels, and Citrine opens your mind to new possibilities in an abundant universe. Place Citrine in the wealth corner of your home—farthest back and at the left as you enter the front door—to draw in abundance. If you tend to procrastinate or are hampered by toxic expectations, Citrine helps you let go of doubt, guilt, fear, or self-pity. It teaches you that what your mind conceives, it achieves.

Poverty consciousness, a mindset of lack, is a base and sacral chakra issue of powerlessness and the inability to create, often instilled by negative parental influences. To transform it into prosperity consciousness, place a Smoky Quartz over the earth star chakra beneath your feet to ground you in the material world and Citrine over your base and sacral chakras to activate your manifestation flow.

It helps you focus on what you want to attract right now and teaches you that when you do what you love, abundance follows. With Citrine in your pocket, you can fulfill your dreams because you recognize that the universe and your soul want you to succeed. This crystal encourages you to be grateful for the small joys of everyday life, sharing life's bounty and taking pleasure in giving. (Note: Citrine is one of the few self-cleaning crystals, but it still benefits from regular purification.)

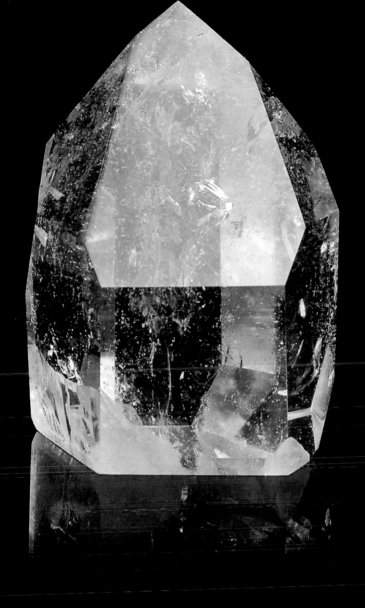

Keep Citrine in your cash drawer
or purse to attract prosperity.

Danburite

- **Chakra correspondences:** Heart, higher heart (thymus), heart seed; activates soul star and stellar gateway
- **Physiological correspondences:** Heart, circulatory system, liver, gallbladder, muscular and motor systems
- **Vibration:** High to exceptionally high

LEGENDARY POWER

Danburite is a powerful heart healer. New finds and alchemicalization processes have raised the crystal's vibrational frequencies, facilitating the connection of the heart and soul star chakras to angelic realms and beyond. Danburite represents the compassionate heart of the universe, the flame of unconditional love that flows through All That Is. It teaches acceptance of things as they are and as they have been.

HEALING POWER

Physically, Danburite may assist the circulation system, detoxify the liver and gallbladder, rectify chronic conditions, alleviate allergies, and strengthen motor and muscular function. Etherically, Danburite dissolves heartbreak and infuses the higher heart and heart seed chakras with unconditional love and acceptance, so that the lightbody can be embodied. Golden Danburite (Agni Gold™) releases psychosomatic and karmic wounds, instilling compassion for yourself and dissolving blockages to spiritual advancement.

TRANSFORMATIONAL POWER

Danburite's power facilitates deep change and profound inner peace. If you have never known love, or are unable to love or forgive yourself, placing Danburite over your heart chakras opens the temple of your inner being, connecting you to unconditional love and the infinite compassion of All That Is. This crystal helps you live in love.

Use Lilac Danburite if grief has blocked the flow of heart energy. It lets you gently release loved ones, safe in the knowledge that you will meet again when your physical existence is over, as a connection of unconditional love is never broken. Golden Danburite connects you to the highest guidance and universal mind, instilling serenity. It facilitates deep karmic and soul healing, cleansing memories and releasing outdated soul imperatives that have prevented your soul's evolution.

Drusy Danburite, with its coating of tiny quartz crystals, amplifies heart energy to an even finer vibration, connecting to archangels and compassionate heart Buddha-energy. This crystal offers the choice of laughing at life no matter how dire your circumstances may be. It is a joyful companion for the terminally ill or deeply depressed as it lifts the spirits to a greater level of insight. The crystal instills patience and aligns you with your soul's timing, rather than the ego's impatience.

Combined with Smoky Quartz, Danburite has a powerful detoxifying and purifying action on the emotions. Aqua Danburite, alchemicalized with pure gold, activates the spiritual gold in your core. This crystal welcomes home soul fragments that were left behind in the heartbreak of past lives and facilitates living from an expanded, accepting, compassionate heart.

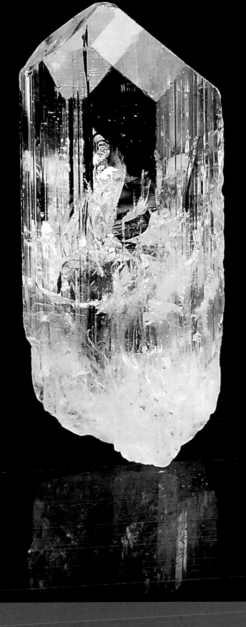

To bring the power of Danburite into your heart, place the crystal over your heart chakra and immerse yourself in warm bathwater for fifteen minutes.

Diamond

- **Chakra correspondences:** Crown
- **Physiological correspondences:** Brain, eyes, metabolism, allergies
- **Vibration:** Earthy and high

LEGENDARY POWER

The hardest substance presently known, Diamond has long been regarded as a symbol of invincibility, what Pliny calls "unconquerable force." Its brilliant faceted form is comparatively recent. In India, Diamonds were believed to be remnants of a pair of cosmic dragons who engaged in a magical sky battle. In fact, the core elements of Diamonds were created not on Earth but in outer space, revealing our cosmic roots. Over eons, through natural processes, the molecules clustered into a single crystal. The ancients clearly had an inkling of this extraterrestrial source.

Black Diamonds traditionally symbolized the void out of which everything formed, and they conveyed the ability to see into the unknown. Pliny believed Diamonds were formed in gold or rock crystal. The early Greek paradoxographer Apollonius marveled that the stone did not grow hot when placed in fire.

In 1867, children in South Africa picked up a Diamond weighing 22.5 karats, and the great diamond rush was on. Diamonds formed part of the paraphernalia of power of many countries. The 195-karat Orloff Diamond, which topped the Russian imperial scepter, was reputed to have been stolen from the eye of an Indian temple statue in Mysore.

Diamond symbolizes purity and eternity, and is the gem for Archangel Metatron. Traditionally, Diamond enhances and amplifies the power of other stones.

HEALING POWER

Pliny believed Diamonds prevailed over poisons, dispelled attacks of "wild distraction," and drove groundless fears from the mind. From ancient times and throughout the Middle Ages, Diamond-infused water was drunk to treat jaundice, gallstones, apoplexy, and fevers. Today, Diamond acts at the mental level to induce clarity and stimulate imagination. It protects against geopathic stress and electromagnetic frequencies.

TRANSFORMATIONAL POWER

A Diamond is dull until faceted and polished; its beauty and brilliance must be revealed slowly with patience and care. The cut is crucial for the finished gemstone's perfection. Unaffected by fire's heat or water's coolness, it symbolizes magical survival through elemental changes. Wearing this crystal provides protection and assists in the assimilation of expanded consciousness and soul evolution. Just as a Diamond has to be "worked," the soul is polished until the refracted light of the inner being creates its own cosmic fire. This gem throws clarity on all that needs to be transmuted and transformed. It is particularly useful for overcoming pride and bringing harmony and accord to the wearer.

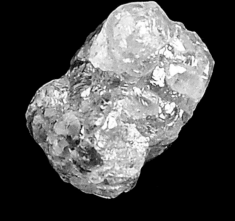

Wear a Diamond, the traditional
gem for engagement rings,
to ensure eternal harmony
between lovers.

Dumortierite

- **Chakra correspondences:** Soma, past life, throat, third eye
- **Physiological correspondences:** Stomach, intestinal tract, cells
- **Vibration:** Earthy

LEGENDARY POWER

First described in 1881, Dumortierite is named after its discoverer, French paleontologist Eugene Dumortier. Its blue color is thought to come from titanium (Rutile). Found in Yuma County, Arizona as fibers embedded in Quartz points, Dumortierite makes an excellent past-life healing tool. Dumortierite is pleochroic and helps you see both sides of an issue.

This stone takes you back to when your soul journey began, connecting you to the innate wisdom of your eternal being. It helps you rescind vows that lie behind poverty, as well as sexual difficulties that arise from past lives of chastity. Dumortierite highlights where your previous soul purpose is no longer appropriate and lets you embrace the lessons your soul set for itself. It also helps you understand why you are encountering certain situations—out of karmic necessity or soul choice? By assisting in cutting ties from the past, it breaks a karmic cycle of dependency on emotions, people, or substances. Use Dumortierite to reprogram cellular memory to release compulsions.

Dumortierite helps you take hold of your destiny. It teaches that karma arises from every thought, word, and deed in the past or present. This stone helps transmute the past so you ascend beyond the vibration of karma into soul choice with right intention. If your vibrations are high and your intention pure, karma no longer has repercussions. But this gentle stone also lets you see why karmic repercussions bounced around for so many lifetimes. It reveals the soul gifts and insights that your higher self gained through such experiences.

HEALING POWER

Dumortierite works best at a subtle level to release psychosomatic and karmic causes of dis-ease but, placed over the abdomen or applied as crystal-infused water, it may ease nausea, cramps, diarrhea, and colic. Slip it under your pillow to aid insomnia. The stone enhances cellular memory and soothes hypersensitivity. Placed over the heart, it calms palpitations and anxiety attacks and, immersed in the bath, soothes sunburn. If you deal with trauma or distress on a daily basis, wear Dumortierite to assist you.

TRANSFORMATIONAL POWER

Practical Dumortierite brings order out of chaos. It reorganizes the body's structure, reprograms your mind, or helps you to re-member your soul. With Dumortierite's support, you gain unshakeable confidence in yourself and your abilities. It teaches that you are never a pawn or a victim, and places you in charge of your own destiny.

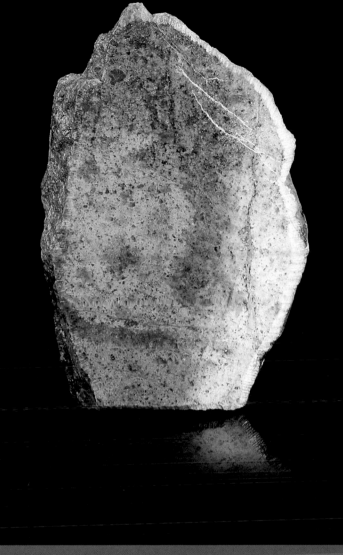

Placed on the soma or past life chakra, Dumortierite aids in exploring previous lifetimes to recognize results of actions, reconnect to karmic skills, and renegotiate contracts.

Elestial Quartz

- **Chakra correspondences:** Earth star and other chakras depending on color
- **Physiological correspondences:** Etheric blueprint, brain cells, pineal gland, all organs according to color
- **Vibration:** High to exceptionally high

LEGENDARY POWER

Elestial Quartz is an anchor for the New Age and a guidebook for the soul's path. This crystal holds pure consciousness within its folds and a new cellular order within its structure. Standing at the energetic interface of the differing vibrations of spirit and matter, it integrates the two. Elestial Quartz rapidly expands your spiritual evolution, preparing the light and physical bodies and stabilizing energy shifts. Its inner doorways open to interdimensions and multidimensions. A powerful catalyst for change, the crystal provides equilibrium during rapid changes, attuning you in each moment.

HEALING POWER

This master healer balances the body and facilitates karmic and etheric purification. Working at multidimensional levels, it restructures energy fields and allows the full potential of DNA to be activated by cellular membranes. Grid Smoky Elestial around your bed to block geopathic stress, prevent nightmares, or relieve depression. Smoky Elestial energetically soaks up ill effects of radiation or chemotherapy and transmutes toxicity into healing dark-light. Place it over the site of pain or trauma.

Rose Elestial heals the physical and etheric hearts and opens the heart seed chakra; Amethyst activates the pineal gland, reattunes the metabolic system and neural pathways, and integrates brain hemispheres.

TRANSFORMATIONAL POWER

The finest transmutor of negative energy, Smoky Elestial grounds grids into everyday reality and anchors healings for the body or Earth. It pulls negative energy out of the environment, transmutes it, and protects the area. In karmic healing, Smoky Elestial helps to reframe the etheric blueprint and ancestral line, transmuting energy back to the beginning of that line so the cellular memory is reprogrammed and power is restored to future generations. In karmic group enmeshment, where similar patterns have repeated lifetime after lifetime, it frees members to choose new pathways.

Amethyst Elestial makes an excellent stabilizing grid, bringing in transmutational forces and creating a calm center where the soul can take refuge as it rides out vibrational shifts. It dissolves addictive patterns and outgrown soul imperatives; combined with Smoky, it aids spirit release work. Clear Elestial Quartz opens the stellar gateway chakra and connects to the highest beings in our universe and beyond. Grid in a star pattern to create sacred space and bring pure consciousness to Earth. Rose Quartz Elestial carries the ray of unconditional love and profound inner change. This compassionate crystal heals ancient heartbreak, dissolves toxic emotions, and sets you free to love again.

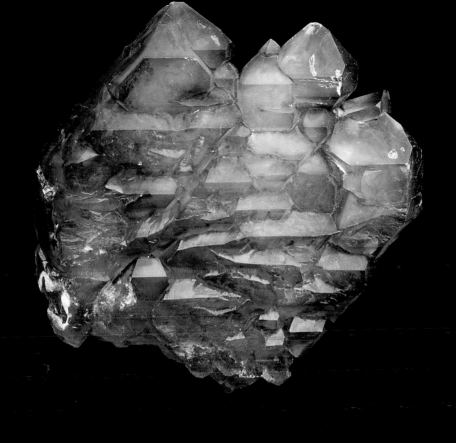

Hold Elestial to understand
the breadth of your soul and its
experiences and to recognize that
inner work, not words or deeds,
propels spiritual evolution.

Emerald

- **Chakra correspondences:** Third eye, heart
- **Physiological correspondences:** Eyes, sinuses, lungs, spine, muscles, heart, pancreas, liver, lymphatic system, malignant conditions
- **Vibration:** Earthy

LEGENDARY POWER

In the seventeenth century, Shakespeare referred to Emerald's power to soothe the eyes: "The deep-green emerald, in whose fresh regard weak sights their sickly radiance do amend." In 1584, Ivan the Terrible believed that Emerald, being of the nature of the rainbow, was an enemy of uncleanness.

Magical legends have long been associated with this rare and precious gemstone. According to Hebrew tradition, serpents that looked on it went blind. Pliny comments on Emerald's use as a magnifying lens and tells us that nothing in nature compared to the stone's intense green: "Neither dim nor shade nor yet the light of a candle, causes them to lose their luster." The seventh-century bishop of Seville, Isidore, reported that Emerald lit up the surrounding area with green light. The Incas prized the crystal highly as representing the green Earth. When taken prisoner by Pizarro in 1532, the last Inca king wore a crown set with 453 Emeralds weighing 1,523 karats (ten ounces). In the Middle Ages, the crystal was placed beneath the tongue to induce prophetic vision. It is linked with Archangel Ophaniel and rules the realm of the Cherubim.

HEALING POWER

The ancient Greek philosopher Theophrastus tells us Emerald was good for eyes, imparting visual clarity. Crystal workers still use Emerald to soothe inflamed eyes and to stimulate sight and insight. The early Persians used it to restore their craftsmen's overtaxed eyesight and to heal stomach and liver ailments. Traditionally, it prevented epilepsy and calmed the spirit, and was said to sweat in the presence of poison. Wearing this stone ensured speedy recovery after illness. It may help to detoxify and stimulate the liver, aiding excretion of poisons from the body via the lymphatic system.

TRANSFORMATIONAL POWER

Emerald symbolizes immortality and rebirth. Whether raw or faceted, this stone provides enormous inspiration on the spiritual path and gives you patience to pass through challenges with equanimity. Promoting friendship and unconditional love, Emerald enhances relationships on all levels, keeping partnerships in harmony. The stone balances the emotional, mental, and spiritual levels, transmuting negativity into positive action. It has long been used to stimulate metaphysical abilities, opening a broader vision that sees beyond the projections of the material world. The power of Emerald was traditionally harnessed to see into the future and to ensure a fortuitous rebirth. (Note: Worn constantly, Emerald can overstimulate.)

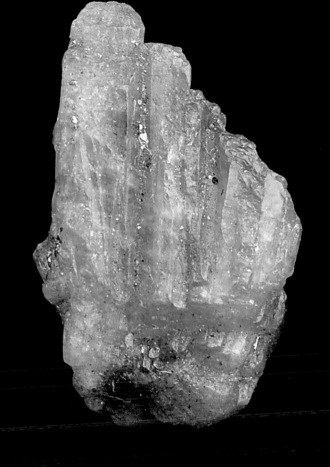

Wear Emerald to attract
successful love—and keep it once
you have found it. This stone has
long been believed to ensure a
happy marriage.

Flint

- **Chakra correspondences:** Earth star, base, sacral, soul star
- **Physiological correspondences:** Jaw, skeleton and joints, reproductive system, skin, cellular and tissue structures, warts, moles, growths, etheric body, energy structure of the physical body
- **Vibration:** Earthy

LEGENDARY POWER

Highly prized in the ancient world, Flint held the essence of fire, that magical element without which life would not exist. From a tiny spark and a whisper of breath, the magical transmutation from rock into flame occurred. Cornelius Agrippa, a fifteenth-century German magician, speaks with awe of *fiery sophus*, Flint stones that created fire and thunderbolts. Flint symbolized the power of the Earth made manifest. Knapped Flint could magically take away life. Around the world, Flint objects were placed in ancient graves, many in pristine condition, indicating their purpose was ritualistic. An acoustic, resonant stone, Flint was believed to open the portal between the worlds and give the soul tools to negotiate the other world. Using this stone ignites the flame of spiritual seeking and hones your soul.

Traditionally, Flint connects to the Green Man, Earth mysteries, the heart of Mother Earth, and power animals. It balances masculine and feminine to create the sacred inner marriage. Use Flint to facilitate rites of passage throughout life. Placed on the earth star, base, and sacral chakras, it forms a shamanic anchor linking your soul to Earth, holding you gently in incarnation and grounding spiritual energies.

HEALING POWER

Flint cleanses the aura and chakras. Two hundred years ago, homeopathic dilutions of Flint treated chronic ulcers or abscesses and "scrofulous troubles of the joints or bones." Flint assists detoxification and pain release, and its shards facilitate etheric surgery and cauterization. Its power heals at emotional, psychological, and energetic levels rather than physical. Metaphorically, it cuts through blockages, past-life ties, and chakra connections that you have outgrown. Taking you deep into yourself, Flint reveals and transmutes underlying causes of depression. It assists you in bringing your shadow's gifts into conscious awareness.

This stone is a powerful Earth healer. When gridded in areas of geopathic stress or energetic disruption, it restores stability, recreating the Earth's energy-meridian matrix.

TRANSFORMATIONAL POWER

Flint stands at the portal between the material and spiritual worlds. By grounding energetic downloads from higher dimensions into the physical body, it creates core stability and restructures information stored in the cells. By cutting away all that no longer serves you, it sets you free from the past. With Flint's assistance you re-member your soul, bringing together fragmentations and lost memories so that you journey home through the portal of your true self. (See Novaculite, page 138.)

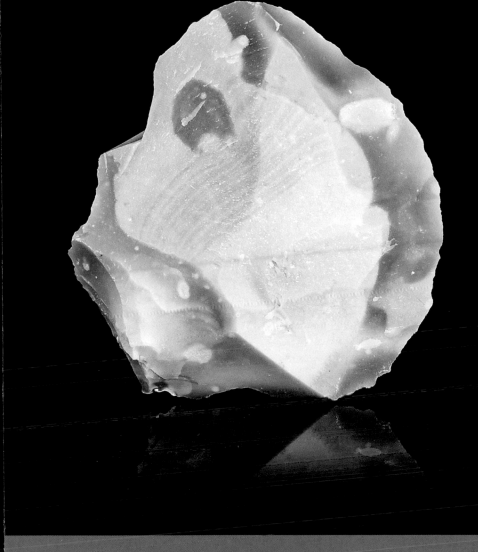

"Comb" the aura a foot or so
out from and around the physical
body with Flint to remove
energetic dis-ease and raise your
energetic frequency.

Fluorite

- **Chakra correspondences:** Heart, higher heart (thymus); cleanses and stabilizes all chakras
- **Physiological correspondences:** Bones, teeth, cells, lungs, DNA, mucus membranes, respiratory and nervous systems, skin, absorption of nutrients
- **Vibration:** Earthy

LEGENDARY POWER

Fluorite is what makes your teeth and bones strong. Although Fluorite was mined in ancient times, little is known about its legendary properties due to problems identifying which stones ancient lapidaries referred to when they spoke of "rainbow hued," "soft banded green," and so on. Cups made of Blue John (a type of Fluorite) dating from ancient Roman times have been found. Known as *fluor spa*, Fluorite was occasionally mentioned in medieval lapidaries, but seems to have been largely overlooked as a magical gem.

The noted gemologist G. F. Kunz describes an early eighteenth-century scientific experiment performed in Germany to demonstrate the effects of crystals on a sensitive person. The psychic chosen was Friederike Hauffe, known as "the seeress of Prevorst." She felt nothing from the first few stones. On coming into contact with Fluorite, however, Hauffe experienced deep muscle relaxation and entered a "somnambulistic state." Today, this energy-stabilizing stone is used to mobilize joints and heal muscle spasm. It is also reputed to enhance trance states and quicken spiritual awakening.

A protective crystal, Fluorite helps you recognize when detrimental external influences are at work and draws off negativity. Place it on your computer to absorb electromagnetic smog. If your energy has become disorganized, Fluorite quickly brings your subtle and physical bodies back into order. It also facilitates information processing.

HEALING POWER

Regarded as a natural antiviral, immune stimulator, and anti-inflammatory agent, Fluorite restores order to the body, particularly the lungs and bones. Crystal workers use it to relieve muscle and joint pain, and to reduce swelling and inflammation associated with arthritis and allied conditions. Placed over the thymus, it counteracts colds and flu. Put it under your pillow to heal night terrors and sleep paralysis and to prevent unwanted out-of-body trips.

Blue Fluorite balances energy, sedating or energizing as required, and focuses brain activity. An effective auric cleanser, Green Fluorite dissipates excess energy and clears emotional trauma. Yellow Fluorite detoxifies the body and the emotions.

TRANSFORMATIONAL POWER

Fluorite helps disorganized people to think straight and get their lives back on track. If you are under any illusions, Fluorite dissolves them so that you can make objective decisions.

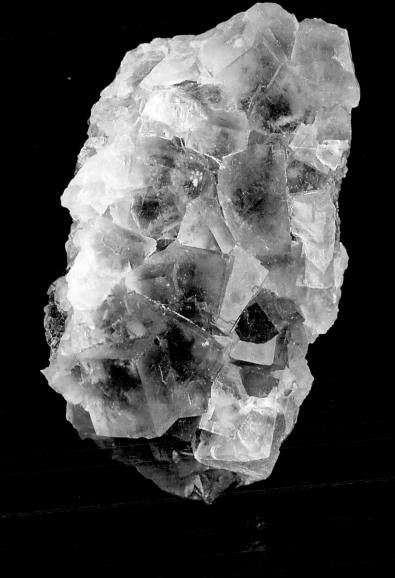

If you need more stability in
your life, mind, body, or emotions,
carry Fluorite at all times to give
you inner strength.

Fire and Ice (Rainbow Quartz)

- **Chakra correspondences:** Cleanses and aligns all chakras; activates soma, soul star, and stellar gateway
- **Physiological correspondences:** Pineal and pituitary glands, endocrine system, reproductive and urinary tracts, the subtle and causal biomagnetic bodies
- **Vibration:** Exceptionally high

LEGENDARY POWER

The bearer of sharp crystal intelligence, this high-vibration Quartz was thermally shocked to create a light bringer that carries cosmic fire within its numerous rainbows. Its innate power fertilizes the Earth and the soul, activating expanded consciousness.

This Quartz contains inner figures that draw on shamanic medicine, and its symbols can be intuitively read for advice regarding soul transformation. You must feel worthy to work with this crystal and be ready to take responsibility for your own emotional, karmic, and ancestral healing—it will assist you, but will not do the work for you or magically dissolve the past. It gently brings up your own "stuff" and supports you during the process of transmutation. A crystal of joy and happiness, resurrection, and rebirth, it links polarities and integrates the full spectrum.

The crystal resonates with the heart chakra of the Andes, the mountain range through which the Earth's kundalini now flows (see Rhodochrosite, page 168). Fire and Ice carries the energy of Buddhist diamond healing and links to Raphael, Archangel of healing. It also connects to ancient Egypt and heals the results of misuse of power from that time.

HEALING POWER

Physically, Fire and Ice works through the pineal and pituitary glands, energetically reconfiguring the endocrine system and neurotransmitters. It may aid the reproductive and urinary tracts in both sexes, activating kundalini to sweep through the kidneys in a cleansing process. It also heals the etheric, causal, and higher spiritual bodies. Fire and Ice opens the central channel and ignites kundalini energy in the lightbody.

TRANSFORMATIONAL POWER

Fire and Ice contains the spirit of pure love. Its purpose is to encompass dark and light within itself to assist in the evolution of the Earth and everything on it. Particularly useful for spiritual manifestation, it has a strong resonance with the law of attraction. A crystal for new beginnings and profound growth, Fire and Ice reveals your soul's purpose and creates a new personal reality. By opening the third eye and assisting kything, it lets you perceive different timelines, endless possibilities, and the beauty of All That Is through its interconnectedness to multirealities and higher dimensions. Fire and Ice recalibrates the resonance of all Quartzes to an expanded level. (Note: Fire and Ice comes from a specific mine in Brazil and has a very high underlying energy. It is not common Crackled Quartz.)

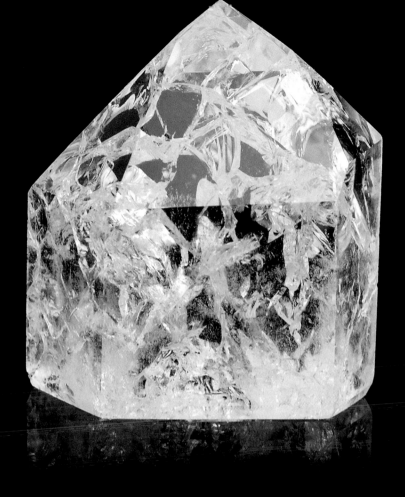

Set your crystal where sunlight
energizes it daily. Each evening,
visualize the sunlight as a beam
passing from the crystal into the
heart of Mother Earth.

Garnet

- **Chakra correspondences:** Base, sacral, heart
- **Physiological correspondences:** Pituitary gland, metabolism, heart, circulation, lungs, liver, spine, cells, DNA, biomagnetic fields, mineral assimilation
- **Vibration:** Earthy to high, depending on type

LEGENDARY POWER

Although the name comes from *granum*, the Latin for granule, in 1885, a Garnet weighing more than 10 pounds (4.5 kg) and measuring 6 inches (15 cm) was found in New York during excavations near Macy's department store. Garnets take many shapes and colors; therefore, this is an extremely versatile group of stones.

Steeped in magical power, Garnet has an ancient history. The Talmud states that Noah's ark was illuminated by a Garnet. Snakes were believed to be guided by Garnets in their foreheads. Crusaders wore the crystal as amulets against accidents. In India, fiery red Garnets were used as bullets because they allegedly had greater killing power.

To dream of a Garnet was considered fortunate, as it indicated the accumulation of riches, but at the same time, the crystal was believed to protect against overindulgence and ensure a balanced life. A crystal of constancy, it was worn by Victorian widows to signify their undying fidelity to their departed spouses; centuries earlier, Garnets were actually buried with the dead. In the language of gems, Garnets indicate loyalty, unchanging affection, and grace, and bring victory to their wearers. The stone of Archangels Zadkiel, Atrugiel, and Michael, it is linked with the angelic realm of Thrones.

HEALING POWER

In medieval times, Garnets were famed for their curative and protective powers, and used to neutralize poison, reduce depression, and calm fever. Under the power of sympathetic magic, red stones were regarded as having anti-inflammatory properties and yellow ones as a sovereign remedy against jaundice. Garnet-infused water aided digestion. Crystal workers today use Garnet to heal heart problems and to revitalize the entire body. The stone also stimulates the metabolic system and assimilation of vital nutrients. Garnet amplifies the energy of other crystals and is particularly useful in regeneration grids.

TRANSFORMATIONAL POWER

Wearing Garnet helps you be faithful to a partner while remaining true to yourself. In ancient times, rounded red Garnets were known as carbuncles, reminding us that they draw festering emotions to the surface for transmutation. With the stone's assistance, you can convert pain, resentment, and dis-ease into well-being. Garnet lets you recognize where you may be sabotaging yourself or resisting change, and it gives you the courage to speak out plus the stamina to maintain your transformation. With Garnet's assistance, you can remain faithful to your purpose. (Note: Garnet is particularly suitable for sensitive people who find Ruby's energy too strong.)

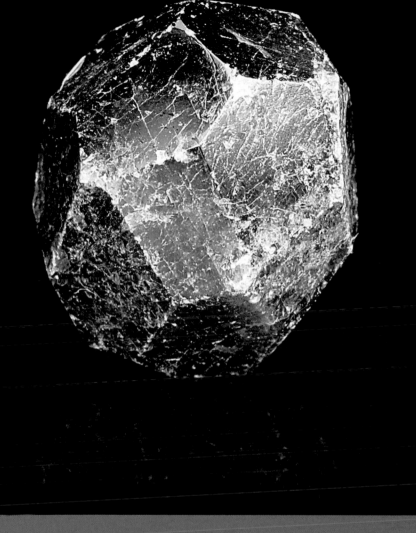

Carry Garnet when it seems
you will never achieve your goal.
It brings hope and the power to
succeed in hopeless situations.

Granite

- **Chakra correspondences:** Soma, past life, earth star, base, sacral
- **Physiological correspondences:** Bones, calcium and mineral assimilation, electrical systems of the body
- **Vibration:** Earthy

LEGENDARY POWER

The ancient Egyptians used powdered Granite to treat white spots of the eye, despite the powder being an irritant. They may have intended to imbue strength and durability, but could have been applying the energetic principle of "like heals like." Granite's high Quartz and Feldspar content produces light-catching crystal specks on its surface. But the magic of Granite lies deeper. Stone circles constructed from Granite have a higher radiation field than the surrounding areas. A powerful current flows through the rock with measurable results. Egyptian Aswan Granite, which has the highest paramagnetic resonance, was believed to harness the power of the sun god Ra and to harmonize the magnetic currents of the surrounding landscape (Texas and Indian Pink Granite have similar but unawakened energy). In the modern-day state of Georgia, Granite "Guidestones" have been astronomically aligned to draw in the Age of Reason.

Granite allows sound to pass through it. Lithophones, as sound rocks are known, seem magical to anyone who witnesses a lump of rock turn into a resonant bell when struck. Such bells are still used as ceremonial instruments in temples in the Far East. In the UK and elsewhere, lithophones situated in wild places were used for shamanic Earth healing rituals.

Many cultures regarded rocks as membranes between the worlds. Cracks in the rocks allowed spirits and shamans to traverse the different realms. Grid Granite to create a sacred space in which to practice magical transformational rituals. Meditating with Aswan Granite helps you reconnect to temple lives and arcane knowledge.

HEALING POWER

Granite has long been used to heal rickets, rheumatism, and infertility. Its stabilizing effect on the human energy field helps realign the subtle bodies with the physical, encouraging electrical activity in cells and stimulating immune response. An excellent sound healer, Granite conveys Qi through its resonant vibrations. Granite grids can neutralize the ill effects of toxic Earth energy lines and reenergize the Earth's magnetic matrix.

TRANSFORMATIONAL POWER

Egyptologist Robert Bauval has described human beings as "star material become conscious" because our bodies contain minerals and elements from outer space. The ancient Egyptians knew about Granite's ability to transform the human energy field to a higher resonance and encouraged humankind to look to the stars for their origins. They utilized Granite to draw the power of the gods to Earth and to assist the Pharaoh on his shamanic journey to the stars. So can you.

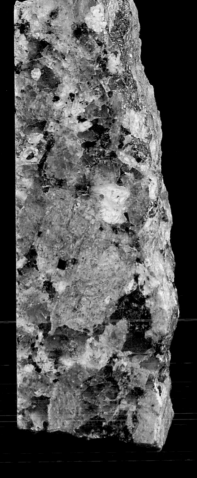

Place a piece of Granite on
the floor at each corner of your
bed to boost the flow of energy
through your body.

Hanksite

- **Chakra correspondences:** Earth star, soma, past life; cleanses and aligns all chakras
- **Physiological correspondences:** Lymphatic system, elimination and detoxifying processes
- **Vibration:** Earthy

LEGENDARY POWER

Hanksite's power draws off toxic energy and catharts the past. The stone comes from the muddy depths of a Californian lake, and symbolizes the wisdom of the soul waiting to be dredged up from the depths of the karmic past. With Hanksite's assistance, you can peel away the past, do the necessary karmic healing, and get down to your core. Halite, a component of Hanksite, is an energetic purifier that stimulates spiritual discernment. Regular sweeps with Halite or Hanksite keep your aura clear and prevent negative entities from attaching.

Hanksite connects to the ancient civilization of Lemuria and brings forward information that has been inaccessible since that time. However, Hanksite warns that this information must be used for the good of all rather than personal gain. Hanksite reveals the damage we are doing to our environment and points out that when we pollute the Earth, we pollute ourselves. If you were involved in power struggles in the past, Hanksite releases these and helps you forgive all concerned. Grid it in toxic places to promote environmental and world healing.

HEALING POWER

Hanksite detoxifies and alleviates fluid retention. It energetically cleanses the lymphatic system and stimulates cellular memory. Hold it to your chest to heal respiratory infections and breathing difficulties caused by inflammation of the mucus membranes.

To facilitate rapid detox, place Hanksite under a healing couch in a Star of David formation with a Smoky Elestial in the center. Other stones may be needed if a catharsis takes place, so this is best done under the supervision of a qualified crystal worker.

Hanksite combines well with Lemurian Seed Crystals and other high-vibration healing stones as it stabilizes healing grids, especially when placed at the feet to draw off negative energy. Cleanse the stone frequently during use. As with Halite, which it contains, Hanksite eventually disintegrates. Bury the remnants in the ground or return them to a body of water to detoxify the environment.

TRANSFORMATIONAL POWER

If you have been carrying a toxic load from previous lifetimes, Hanksite transmutes destructive and blocked emotions into forgiveness and regeneration. It helps you retrieve parts of your soul left in other lifetimes or dimensions, then assists in reintegrating them, purifying the parts as they are returned. Just as Hanksite aids your soul's renewal, it also regenerates the Earth, and lets you apply ancient solutions to modern problems.

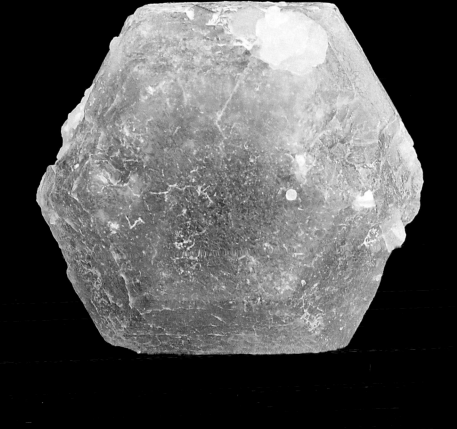

Place Hanksite that has not been treated with oil to maintain its crystal integrity in bathwater or under the shower to cleanse your aura.

Healer's Gold™

- **Chakra correspondences:** Earth star, base, sacral, higher heart (thymus), past life
- **Physiological correspondences:** Cellular structures, energetic meridians, immune system, physical vitality, blood, bones, DNA, digestive tract, circulatory and respiratory systems
- **Vibration:** Earthy and high

LEGENDARY POWER

Healer's Gold is a powerful, synergistic combination of Iron Pyrite and Magnetite, which come under Mars's influence and so tend to speed up things. At a vibrational level, the stone brings core issues to the surface for resolution.

Magnetite has a strong positive-negative polarity and can be used for magnet therapy or Earth healing. Iron Pyrite protects the subtle bodies, deflecting harmful energies and negative thoughts. The combination prevents energy leakage from the auric body and helps to ground high-frequency energies into the physical body and the Earth.

Healer's Gold aids healers whose energy drops during the healing process, which indicates that the healer is giving away personal life energy or taking in negative energy from the patient. Healer's Gold teaches you to work at the vibrational interface between personal energy fields, passing on universal healing energy and sending negativity to the stone for transmutation.

Healer's Gold also provides a useful energetic shield to guard against electromagnetic pollution or other negative energies in the external world. Because it contains iron, it also protects you from the harmful intentions of others. The synergistic properties of Magnetite and Pyrite block negative energies at the interface, returning them to the source so that understanding can be reached. Through sympathetic magic, the combination also transmutes psychic attacks.

HEALING POWER

Healer's Gold boosts the energy systems of both healer and recipient, and enhances the flow of Qi throughout both people's bodies. The perfect stone for dis-eases affecting the immune system, its powerful balancing ability energetically sedates or stimulates as appropriate—especially if the body is trying too hard to heal itself, resulting in inflammation or fever. Healer's Gold speeds recovery from chronic illness and renews vitality during convalescence. It moves sluggish energy through blocked meridians, bringing the body back into harmony. For sports injuries, pass Healer's Gold over the damaged site to increase blood flow, draw out pain, relax muscles, and stabilize tendons and bones.

TRANSFORMATIONAL POWER

The power of Healer's Gold to transmute negative energies and kick-start stuck situations is much stronger than that of its individual components. Excellent for overcoming psychological despair when an illness or situation does not appear to be shifting, the stone instills confidence and feelings of well-being. If you've experienced an abusive past, Healer's Gold helps you find the gold in the core of your being. Lemurian Jade is energetically similar to Healer's Gold.

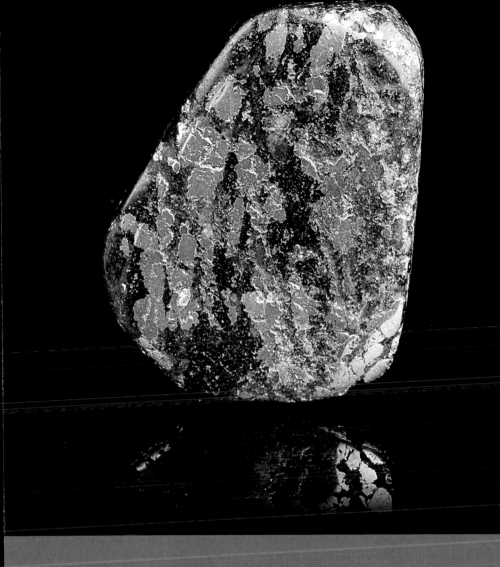

Wear Healer's Gold to create
a magnetic shield to prevent
depletion or invasion of your
personal energetic space.

Hematite

- **Chakra correspondences:** Earth star, base, past life, crown
- **Physiological correspondences:** hemoglobin, formation of red blood cells, circulation, absorption of iron, liver, triple heater meridian, temperature regulation, kidneys, blood-rich organs
- **Vibration:** Earthy; Specularite (Specular Hematite) and Hematite with Rutile have higher vibrations

LEGENDARY POWER

According to Greek myth, Hematite was created when Saturn killed his father, the tyrannical god Uranus. This ancient "cycle myth" describes the destruction of the old to make way for the new. Hematite was often called *bloodstone* because it looked like blood when pulverized or heated. When polished, magnetic red Hematite magically becomes silver and has a noticeable attraction or repulsion effect depending on the polarities.

In the *Alexander Romance*, an early mythobiography of Alexander the Great, the magician Nectanebo cast a crystal birth chart to foretell Alexander's conception. Hematite represented the planet Mars. The act set in motion a deception by which Nectanebo pretended to be the sun god Amon Ra and impregnated the Queen. Thus, the stone has always had a reputation for aiding deception or manipulators to gain advantage.

Pliny tells us the Mesopotamians believed Hematite cured diseases of the eyes and liver. As a talisman in lawsuits, it brought about favorable outcomes, although not necessarily just ones. Pliny also writes that the Babylonians made a paste out of Hematite, which when smeared on warriors, ensured success in battle—not surprisingly, as the stone was closely associated with Mars, the god of war.

HEALING POWER

One of the earliest Mesopotamian healing remedies uses Hematite to cool the blood. The 3,500-year-old Egyptian *Ebers Papyrus* recommends using it to control bleeding and reduce inflammation. In ancient Egypt, Hematite was powdered and mixed with honey and oil to treat stomach ailments. Al Biruni suggests using Hematite for palsy and paralysis, especially facial. Crystal workers today still employ Hematite for ailments connected to blood, including anemia, hemorrhage, and circulatory problems. The stone also draws off heat from the body in conditions such as inflammation and arthritis. A powerfully *yang* (masculine) stone, it balances *yin* (feminine) energy.

Useful for past-life healings that involve war, wounds, and bloodshed, this powerful stone also assists in overcoming addictions rooted in emotional cravings or unfulfilled desires. Hold Hematite to ground the soul back into your body after journeying or spiritual work.

TRANSFORMATIONAL POWER

This stone's power overcomes weakness or timidity of any kind and enhances self-esteem. Wearing it strengthens personal power and magnetism, bringing out your latent charisma.

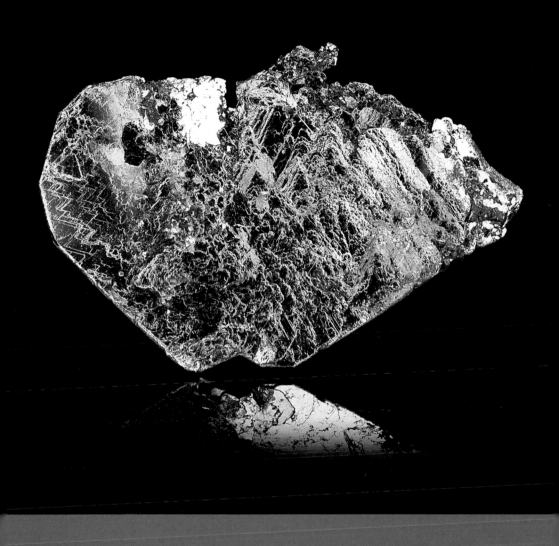

Carry Hematite in your pocket to create a power shield that protects you from electromagnetic smog and geopathic, physical, or mental stress.

Herkimer Diamond

- **Chakra correspondences:** All
- **Physiological correspondences:** Metabolism and detoxification systems, neural pathways, cellular structure, DNA
- **Vibration:** High to exceptionally high

LEGENDARY POWER

Herkimer Diamond is a form of Quartz that often contains oil, carbon, or mineral inclusions that add to the stone's magical properties. One of the oldest Quartzes, it slowly formed underwater hundreds of millions of years ago and holds the wisdom of the ages in its crystalline depths. Formed as individual crystals within a matrix, Herkimers are double-terminated. Therefore, they help both to break old patterns and to retrieve and reintegrate parts of the soul that fragmented in other lives.

Herkimers unite body, mind, spirit, multidimensions, and consciousness into an integrated whole. They work well as a multidimensional information highway. A powerful agent of transmutation and purification, Herkimer Diamond protects against electromagnetic smog and geomagnetic pollution. Gridded around an area of environmental disharmony, it restores equilibrium.

HEALING POWER

Herkimers are effective energy detoxifiers, whether used in grids or placed on the chakras. Grid Herkimer Diamonds around your bed to overcome insomnia caused by environmental factors. By drawing energy into your body to create new neural pathways and facilitate cellular informational downloads, the crystal restructures etheric DNA, reattuning your metabolism to a higher frequency. Smoky Herkimers are effective for environmental healing and for stabilizing energies. Golden Enhydro Herkimers, which contain bubbles of oil inside, effect profound emotional healing. All Herkimers energize water into a potent healing elixir. Under the direction of an experienced crystal therapist, Herkimers can inspire powerful soul healing.

TRANSFORMATIONAL POWER

Herkimers transform the way you see the world. They aid you in creating within the physical body new neural pathways that connect to the lightbody and to All That Is to manifest your spiritual potential on Earth. Herkimer attunes you to a much higher reality and accelerates your spiritual growth, so you become coherent at every level of being.

Amethyst Herkimer is rare, but has an exceptionally high vibration that aligns the incarnated portion of your soul with that which exists in other dimensions. A powerful shield for the soul when journeying through interdimensional realms, it creates the highest spiritual connections. Yellow ("Citrine") Herkimer transmutes poverty consciousness from past-life vows into prosperity consciousness that attracts abundance to your soul. Blue Herkimer infused with Boulangerite brings a new sense of vision. This beautiful but extremely rare crystal helps you explore the inner reaches of your self and reconnect to your soul knowing. (Note: Herkimers combine particularly well with Shungite for environmental healing.)

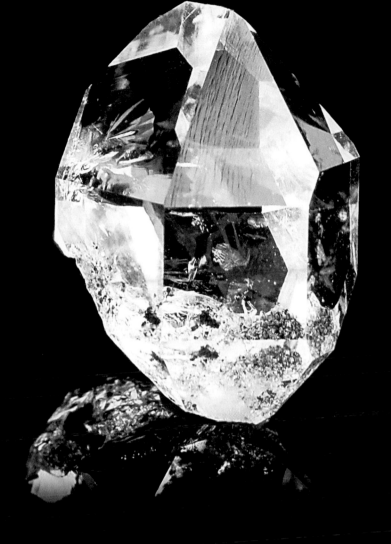

Place a Herkimer on your
third eye to enhance telepathic
communication and spiritual
vision, and attune you to the
highest source of soul guidance.

Idocrase (Vesuvianite)

- **Chakra correspondences:** Third eye, heart
- **Physiological correspondences:** Teeth, bones, sense of smell, assimilation of nutrients
- **Vibration:** Earthy to high

LEGENDARY POWER

In crystal lore, Idocrase is known as Vesuvianite as it was first found in rocks thrown out of Mount Vesuvius. This powerful crystal helps you follow your heart's desire, rather than that of your ego or karma.

Karmic debts need not be paid to those with whom they arose, but can be mitigated by service given as an act of soul intention. Idocrase lets you take a new direction of service to your fellow beings, making nonspecific restitution and assisting the evolution of the whole. If nothing more can be achieved through a karmic connection, Idocrase facilitates graceful release. When forgiving those with whom you have karma, you release your bond to the karmic wheel. Idocrase helps you embrace life circumstances that arose from karmic necessity or your soul's choice. It also assists you in giving service willingly to those who are learning compassion or empathy through situations of abuse, trauma, or alienation.

Useful for healing the past—especially one constrained by external circumstances, guilt, or your own mental beliefs—Idocrase sets your soul free to pursue a new pathway. It releases fear so you can stand up for what is right. By gently dissolving toxic emotions, such as anger or guilt, Idocrase helps you build an energetically stable inner core. Idocrase relates to Archangel Zadkiel.

HEALING POWER

Under the power of sympathetic magic, Idocrase's calcium-magnesium formula strengthens bones and tooth enamel. It energetically assists the assimilation of nutrients and vitamins. Sniffing up Idocrase-infused water (a variation of an ancient yogic tradition that uses saltwater) may restore your sense of smell.

TRANSFORMATIONAL POWER

Idocrase builds a bridge to the higher self, enabling it to offer information to the soul in incarnation. By suspending judgment and clearing old beliefs and ingrained patterns, the stone opens your mind to universal wisdom. It is especially helpful in clearing beliefs instilled by others or where paying lip service to others' beliefs blocks greater insight.

This powerful crystal stimulates your urge to learn about the multidimensions that surround the physical world. It helps disconnect the ego's drive to be powerful and successful in the outer world, turning your attention to inner growth and attuning your will to your higher self. The higher self carries knowledge of why your soul is in incarnation at this time. When you suspend judgment of your karma or that of others, you recognize the universal justice and gifts in all you experience.

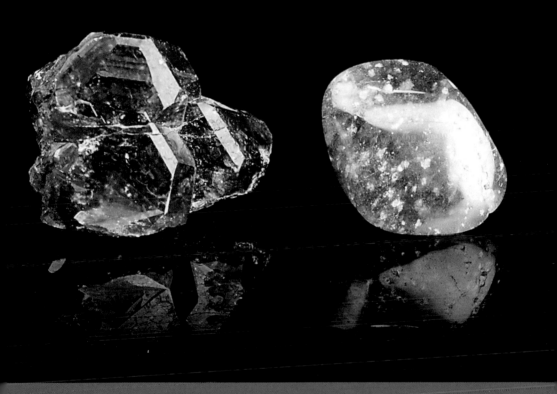

Meditate with Idocrase to identify and release outmoded soul imperatives and to recognize the ultimate fairness of karmic justice.

Iolite

- **Chakra correspondences:** Third eye, soma; aligns all chakras
- **Physiological correspondences:** Arteries, liver, pituitary gland, detoxification and elimination processes, respiratory system
- **Vibration:** High

LEGENDARY POWER

The name *Iolite* derives from the Greek *Ios*, meaning violet. It is known as the water sapphire because when you look into the stone, it resembles tranquil water. Iolite's beautiful colors vary depending on the direction from which you view the stone. This three-way pleochroism reflects the vision and inner knowledge that the crystal contains. Placed on the third eye or soma chakra, Iolite stimulates clairvoyance and kything. By enhancing visualization, it can take you journeying through other realms or lifetimes.

Iolite contains the power of insight and carries a dynamic hologram of soul knowing. Perception and insight work at different levels. Everyday awareness perceives the external world and the signals it gives off. Yet behavior is unconsciously driven by emotional awareness. This instinctive awareness is mediated through the oldest part of the brain, its stem. The neural programming connected to it includes the fight-or-flight mechanism.

At this level, reality is viewed as three-dimensional. Illusions and misunderstandings occur, based on what you have been conditioned to expect or on your inner constitutional state. Iolite expands metaphysical perception and heightens intuition. This way of experiencing the world aligns intention and perception, going beyond the bounds of consensual reality into a wider awareness of the physical and nonphysical worlds.

Iolite may be the "compass crystal" the Vikings used to navigate during sea voyages. It provides an excellent spiritual compass, too. Iolite is attributed to Archangels Gabriel, the angel of vision, and Michael, the spiritual warrior.

HEALING POWER

Iolite contains magnesium and iron, and its homeopathic magic strengthens your constitution at every level. With its powerful electrical charge, the crystal reenergizes the auric field, detoxifies the physical body, and may prevent bacteria from reproducing and dissolve cholesterol in the arteries. It stimulates the pituitary gland and regulates metabolism. Crystal workers use Iolite to heal the sinuses and respiratory system, and to heal fevers and malaria. This crystal balances the flow of yin and yang within the energy meridians, bringing the body to optimum health.

TRANSFORMATIONAL POWER

Use Iolite if you are caught up in codependent relationships—it encourages taking responsibility for yourself. By stimulating insights into the reasons behind addictions of all kinds, the stone helps release you from the expectations of others and lets you express your true self. With Iolite's ability to create perceptive inner vision and reconnect to your deepest knowing, you will live in a different world.

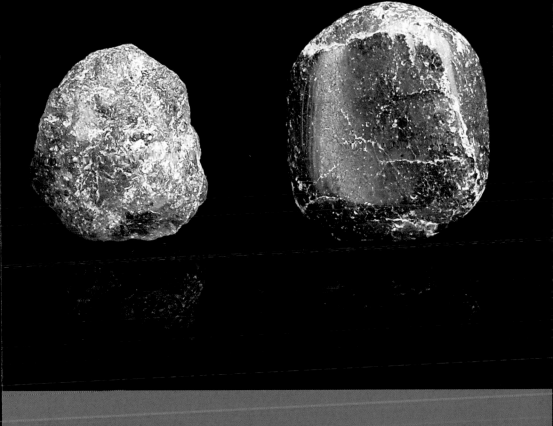

Meditate with Iolite on your
third eye to experience direct
perception of All That Is and to
log into the holographic nature of
universal mind.

Jade

- **Chakra correspondences:** Soma, third eye, solar plexus, heart; varies according to color
- **Physiological correspondences:** Kidneys, adrenal glands, spleen, hips, skeletal and filtration systems, fluid balance
- **Vibration:** Earthy to high, depending on color

LEGENDARY POWER

The Chinese considered Jade the most precious gem as it held five great virtues— wisdom, justice, modesty, courage, and purity—plus five happinesses—wealth, old age, health, natural death, and love of virtue. They inserted Jade into high-status corpses to delay decomposition, but this may have had ritualistic meaning given its connection to purity and vitality of the soul. In New Zealand, the Maori wore "greenstone" talismans to ensure long life and fertility.

The Aztecs prized Jade for its healing properties and connection to their gods. Its name derives from the Spanish *piedra de hijada*, meaning "stone of the loins or flank." The Spanish named it Jade when they conquered South America. The indigenous people believed the stone cured kidney diseases. The English explorer Sir Walter Raleigh also encountered Jade on his travels and used it for "spleene stones" and "the stone" (gallstones).

A stone of weather magic, Jade was believed in antiquity to call up wind, rain, snow, or mist, and to have power over the Earth's elements. Muslims wore Jade amulets to protect against "injury and annoyance."

This stone signifies wisdom gathered in tranquility; it aids meditation and stress release. Placed on your forehead or under your pillow, it induces insightful dreams and helps you understand their meanings. In the language of crystals, Jade symbolizes good fortune and protection.

HEALING POWER

The early Chinese thought Jade was a cleansing cure-all. Powdered and mixed with water, it prolonged life, prevented fatigue, and delayed decomposition or formation of pus. Jade healed asthma and diseases of the blood, and it is still used for this purpose today. In the Middle Ages, Jade assisted childbirth, reduced palpitations, and relieved dropsy. Modern crystal workers use it to detoxify the kidneys and adrenals, and to energetically restructure cells. Jade is a powerful muscle relaxant. Place it gently over the site to encourage healing of stitches and abrasions.

TRANSFORMATIONAL POWER

Jade is an excellent stone for restoring your soul's purity and for nurturing you while in incarnation. Blue Jade brings serenity and aids people who are overwhelmed by their life situations. Brown Jade connects to the supportive energy of the Earth. Delicate Lavender Jade helps heal emotional trauma and takes you to a higher level of relationship with yourself and others. Yellow Jade gently energizes, but Orange and Red are powerfully invigorating, enhancing vitality and igniting passion for life. White Jade is the ultimate symbol of purity.

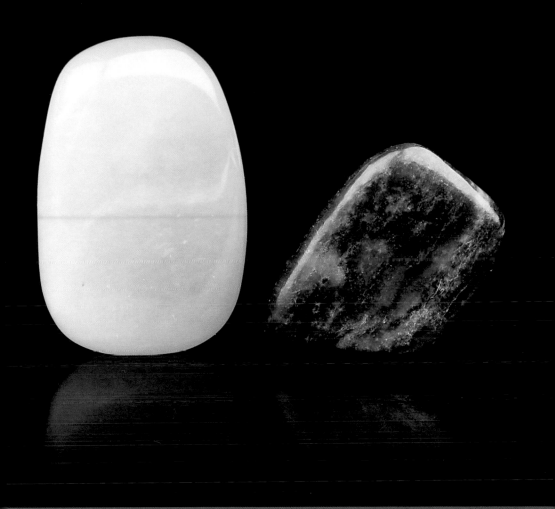

Hold Jade over your solar plexus for a
few minutes each day to stabilize your
psyche and emotions and help you
live harmoniously on the Earth.

Jasper

- **Chakra correspondences:** Earth star, base, sacral, solar plexus, throat (according to color); aligns all chakras
- **Physiological correspondences:** Circulation, digestion, sexual function, reproductive organs, liver, mineral assimilation
- **Vibration:** Earthy

LEGENDARY POWER

In a Mesopotamian creation legend, the god Marduk (Jupiter) formed three "heavens" or spheres above the Earth, the lower one created from Jasper. On it, he drew the constellations. Around 350 B.C.E., the Greek poet Posidippus called the stone "misty Jasper, the ethereal stone," echoing this belief.

The ancient Egyptians associated it with the menstrual blood of the goddess Isis; the stone assisted pregnant women and increased lactation. Early lapidaries say Jasper offered protection against disease and energized the body. Believed to protect its owner from drowning, a Jasper amulet also kept spiders and scorpions at bay. It guarded against sorrow and relieved drought. The fourth-century B.C.E. *Lithica* stated, "Whoe'er the polished grass-green jasper wears his parched globe they'll satiate with rain."

Jasper symbolizes nurturing, courage, and wisdom. The early Christian lapidary of Epiphanius, Bishop of Salamis in Cyprus, credited green Jasper with the power to drive away evil fantasies. In fifteenth-century German High Magic, it acted against "offensive imaginings," and in the sixteenth century, it expelled "noxious phantasms." Today, we would call these paranoid delusions and entity attachments. Jasper helps you cope if you feel overwhelmed by unpleasant nightmares or beset by evil entities.

Jasper is a stone of Archangels Haniel and Sandalphon, ruling the Angelic Principalities.

HEALING POWER

Traditionally, Jasper healed dis-eases of the stomach, lungs, and chest. According to Cornelius Agrippa and Al Biruni, it facilitated birth. A 1587 Dutch lapidary reported that Jasper staunched blood and regulated the pulse. The stone was said to increase fertility and creativity, overcoming impotence.

Wear Jasper to ameliorate stress and induce tranquility. Brown and Picture Jasper facilitate karmic healing, draw out ancient toxins, and boost the immune system. Yellow Jasper encourages emotional detoxification and calms digestive processes.

TRANSFORMATIONAL POWER

A stone of courage, Jasper helps you be honest with yourself when facing problems. It lets you move forward assertively, rather than aggressively. If you have been selfish or self-centered, holding Jasper reminds you to work harmoniously with others.

Green Jasper balances obsessive tendencies and restores harmony. Purple Jasper eliminates contradictions and paradoxes. Yellow Jasper offers protection during out-of-body journeys. If you have difficulty keeping your feet on the ground, carry Brecciated Jasper to ground you physically and spiritually. Meditating with Rainforest Jasper renews your contact with nature. If you have been led astray spiritually, it returns you to your true path. (See Poppy Jasper, page 158.)

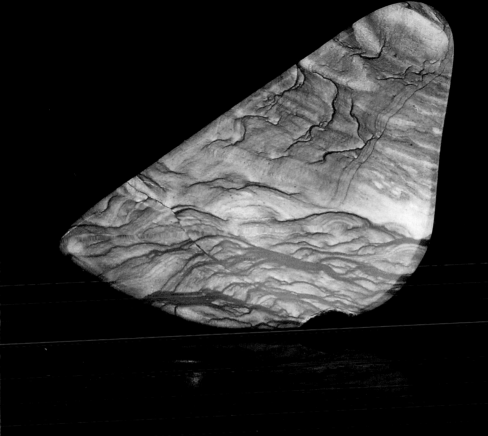

Place Jasper on the base chakra
to stabilize and energize your
physical body. Laid over each
chakra in turn, it cleanses, boosts,
and realigns energy.

Kunzite (Spodumene)

- **Chakra correspondences:** Heart, higher heart (thymus), heart seed, throat, third eye
- **Physiological correspondences:** Brain chemistry, circulatory system and heart, thymus, immune system, etheric bodies
- **Vibration:** High

LEGENDARY POWER

Early in the twentieth century, American gemologist G. F. Kunz named lilac-pink Kunzite after himself; the green form was named Hiddenite after W. E. Hidden, who had found it earlier in North Carolina. Kunz noted its unusual property of absorbing light and then giving it out in the darkness. He suggests this is due to minute quantities of manganese or uranium salts in its composition, which absorb the ultraviolet spectrum. A dichroic crystal, its color changes in different lights. You literally see things in a different light with Kunzite.

Kunzite exemplifies the principle by which a minute amount of a substance vibrationally assists the condition that in a larger dose it causes. The stone contains lithium, traditionally used to stabilize bipolar disorder. However, lithium must be closely monitored—an overdose is highly toxic and depresses the brain. Crystal workers heal psychiatric disorders, emotional stress, and depression with Kunzite. The crystal or Kunzite-infused water conveys vibrational information from the traces of lithium and aluminum in the stone to the recipient. Kunzite also acts as a "radionic witness," a surrogate for a person being healed at a distance. Use it to cleanse and shield your auric bodies from unwanted influences.

Kunzite resonates with the heart and heart chakra chambers. Placed over the heart seed chakra, Kunzite opens and activates the temple of the inner self. It assists in remembering your soul and reveals the purpose of incarnation. Placed on the higher heart chakra, it brings the heart, throat, and third eye chakras into alignment to facilitate self-expression.

HEALING POWER

In modern crystal work, Kunzite is used for emotional and mental healing by placing the crystal over appropriate chakras, as a grid around the body, or as Kunzite-infused water. Kept in the pocket, placed on the solar plexus, or worn around the neck, it quickly calms panic attacks or chronic anxiety. To heal heartache or to support the circulatory system, place it over the heart chakra; put it over the thymus to energetically strengthen the immune system. Use Kunzite after receiving anesthesia to remove vibrational residue from the etheric body.

TRANSFORMATIONAL POWER

Kunzite sends out loving thoughts and supports you in selfless service to humanity. Lilac Kunzite acts as a celestial doorway and assists transitions; Hiddenite facilitates the transfer of knowledge from the higher mind. It helps people who put on a brave face, encouraging them to accept support from others. Heart, mind, and soul become tranquil under Kunzite's calming influence.

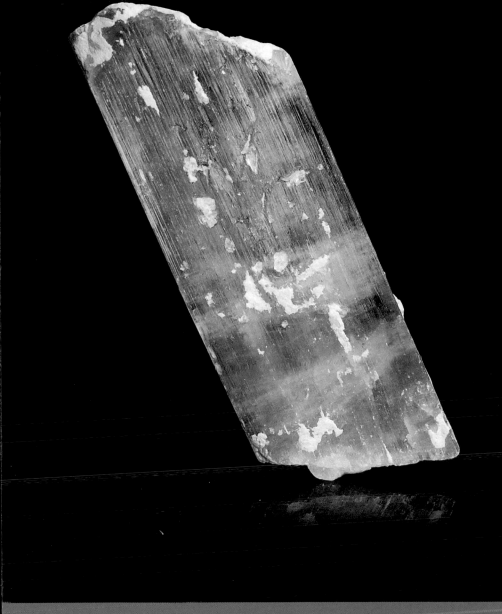

To resolve a conflict with yourself
or someone else, hold Kunzite and
picture its gentle energy radiating
around you and out into the world.

Labradorite

- **Chakra correspondences:** Higher heart (thymus), throat, third eye, soma; purifies, aligns, and protects all chakras
- **Physiological correspondences:** Eyes, brain, neurotransmitters, spleen, stomach, liver, adrenal glands, gallbladder, blood pressure, metabolic and hormonal systems
- **Vibration:** High to extremely high, depending on type

LEGENDARY POWER

Labradorite is a stone of exceptional spiritual power. Helping to prepare the physical body for the expansion process, it anchors the lightbody in place and connects to the highest energies in the universe as it opens spiritual vision. Standing at the vibrational junction of spirit and matter, protective Labradorite creates an interface that facilitates metaphysical working. It enables you to monitor what is going on in another energy field without taking on conditions from that field or entering it. By blocking other people's projections, Labradorite removes mental or other hooks from your aura. It also prevents energy leakage or vampirization by a discarnate spirit.

This stone's intuitive wisdom balances analysis and rationality with inner *knowing* and perceptive insight. Labradorite goes to the core of a matter and brings up suppressed issues for resolution (for which other crystals may be needed). It banishes fear, especially fear caused by a subconscious memory of having suffered in past lives because you were psychic.

HEALING POWER

Place Labradorite on your third eye to heal eye dis-eases and migraines that arise from blocked psychic power. At a physical level, Labradorite laid in the hollow in the back of the skull may regulate metabolism and hormonal balance and relieve PMS. Crystal healers use it to heal inflammatory conditions, such as rheumatism or gout. Worn over the higher heart chakra, it protects against colds and may lower blood pressure. Labradorite acts as a witness during distant radionic treatment.

TRANSFORMATIONAL POWER

This powerful stone opens spiritual pathways and attunes you to your soul's purpose in incarnating. Labradorite connects you with the greater part of your soul that is outside incarnation so you receive guidance from that source.

Golden-Yellow Labradorite (Bytownite) activates the third eye and lets you access the highest levels of consciousness; it facilitates metaphysical working of all kinds. If you are inappropriately dependent on someone or something, Bytownite helps you detach and stand in your own power.

Spectrolite's extremely fine resonance protects the soul no matter where it journeys. The crystal also detaches thought forms from the aura. Particularly useful if you have elected to evolve through challenging life conditions, it connects you to your highest self's guidance and support. Violet Hypersthene (Velvet Labradorite) brings anger and emotional toxicity to the surface for transmutation and assists you in facing your deepest fears. It is an excellent companion for lower-world journeying.

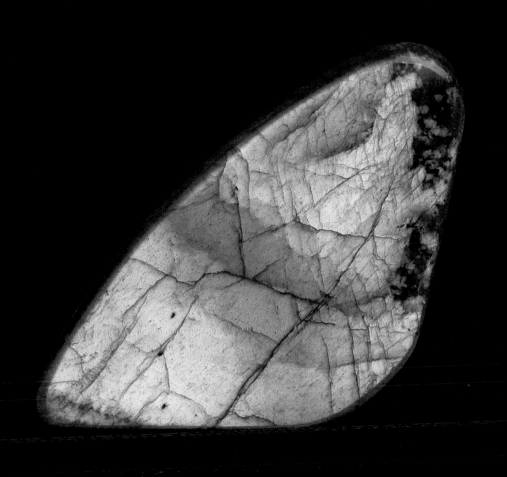

Held over the crown chakra,
Labradorite aligns and recalibrates
the physical and subtle etheric
bodies to higher-frequency encrgy
to shield you from detrimental
external influences.

Lapis Lazuli

- **Chakra correspondences:** Throat, third eye, soma, crown
- **Physiological correspondences:** Immune system, eyes, nervous and respiratory systems, bone marrow, throat, thyroid gland, larynx, ears, blood
- **Vibration:** High

LEGENDARY POWER

Lapis Lazuli represented the night sky and the power of the gods to the ancient Egyptians. *The Primeval Ocean* tells us, "Lapis is the god and the god is Lapis," and the stone symbolizes cosmic correspondence. What is below is a reflection of what is above, carrying the same powers and sharing the same energetic signature.

Transported from a remote mine in Afghanistan, Lapis symbolized royal power for eons. In Mesopotamian legend, the goddess Inanna (Venus) wore her Lapis regalia when she went into the underworld to comfort her sister-goddess whose husband had died:

> *From the Great Above the goddess opened her ear to the Great Below . . .*
> *Inanna abandoned heaven and earth to descend to the underworld . . .*
> *She tied the small lapis beads around her neck.*
> *Let the double strand of beads fall to her breast . . .*
> *And took the lapis measuring rod and line in her hand.*

The Lapis rod measured the natural world's cycles, and Inanna's beads symbolized eternal life. In the underworld, she was stripped, flayed, and hung on a peg. We can interpret this myth in many ways. Pragmatically, it depicts seasonal changes or the temporary disappearance of Venus as it transforms from the evening to the morning star. Psychologically, it represents the death of the ego. Spiritually, it describes the soul's journey to Earth, an initiation ritual of dying to the old self, or even a basic chakra cleansing as Inanna is stripped of seven items. The myth signifies that rebirth follows death and the spirit can be transformed—a process facilitated by Lapis Lazuli, which stores the energy of the core self. Lapis is the stone of Archangel Michael.

HEALING POWER

In ancient Egyptian medicine, Lapis enhanced the expectation of a cure; today we recognize this as the "placebo effect," which encourages healing. The *Ebers Papyrus* says Lapis cured eye dis-eases and prevented miscarriage. The Alfonso lapidary also says powdered Lapis was applied to the eyes or drunk as a potion to purge "thick humors" and melancholy. It was also given as a remedy for bladder pain and to regulate menstrual courses. Crystal workers today utilize its copper-based power to alleviate pain, induce detoxification, lower blood pressure, and stimulate the immune system.

TRANSFORMATIONAL POWER

Lapis's high electrical conductivity channels the pureness of being, sensitizing you to higher vibrations. By transmuting mental and emotional blockages, Lapis sets your soul free to express itself fully.

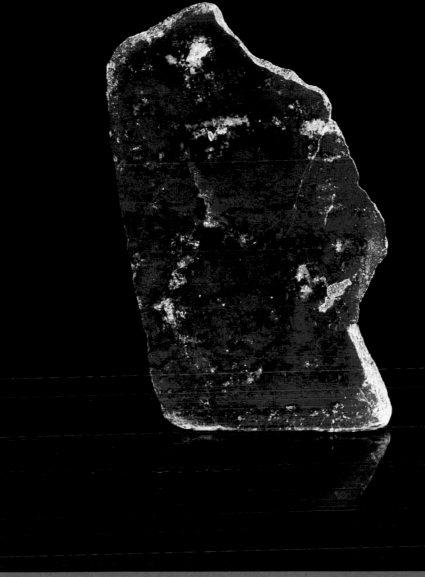

Meditate with Lapis to stimulate
your third eye, facilitate
metaphysical sight, and access
inner truth. With this stone, you
are literally in heaven on Earth.

Lemurian Seed

- **Chakra correspondences:** Cleanses and activates all chakras and the central channel
- **Physiological correspondences:** Subtle energy bodies
- **Vibration:** Exceptionally high

LEGENDARY POWER

Lemurian Seed instigates a profound vibrational shift in the Earth and everything upon it. Lemurians were discovered lying loose in a bed of sand, rather than being attached to a matrix as crystals usually are. Originally found in Brazil, they now have manifested elsewhere in the world. Crystal lore says a Lemurian civilization left them, encoded with the vibrational information required to open a New Age on Earth at the present time.

A symbol of equality and personal power, Lemurians teach that we are multi-dimensional and interdimensional beings. By piercing our illusion of separateness from the rest of the cosmos and dissolving the boundaries of time, these crystals help you to rectify personal misuse of power in the past and remove karmic debris so you can regain inner perfection.

Lemurians open a portal that brings ancient wisdom—personal, collective, and cosmic—back into conscious awareness. They demonstrate that time is an illusion of the material plane, and take you into the multidimensions of being. Lemurians activate the higher resonance of each chakra. However, they also alert you to the dangers of spiritual egoism. They warn against feeling spiritually superior and arrogantly telling people what to do. Instead, they encourage you to simply *be* in each moment and attend to your own evolution.

HEALING POWER

These powerful healing crystals work at a multidimensional level to remove all that is dis-eased or blocked within the physical and subtle energy bodies, chakras, and meridians. By attuning the central channel that connects the chakras, they draw subtle Earth energy up from the earth star and bring cosmic energy down through the crown chakra to unite at the heart, opening interdimensional consciousness within the body. Lemurians realign the physical and subtle bodies and attune neural pathways to higher frequencies.

TRANSFORMATIONAL POWER

Lemurians teach that healing is a re-membering of your soul. Everyone must personally attend to dissolving the destructive emotional patterns, energy blockages, and mental beliefs that prevent an infusion of light into the physical level of being. Lemurians demonstrate that we cocreate our own realities with every thought, word, and deed. They teach you to become creative in the higher dimensions, not merely by holding positive thoughts in the outer world, but by taking this way of being deep into inner awareness. With this crystal, you explore the whole range of consciousness, so you know what it is to be a truly awakened soul.

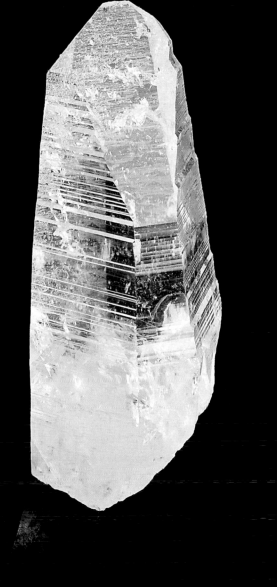

Gently stroke Lemurian's
horizontal striations from bottom
to top to read the Lemurian or
Atlantean past. Or, ascend them like
a ladder to expanded consciousness.

Malachite

- **Chakra correspondences:** Earth, base, sacral, heart, solar plexus
- **Physiological correspondences:** Urogenital tract, liver, gallbladder, pancreas, bones, DNA, tissue, spleen, parathyroid gland, cellular structures, and circulatory, lymphatic, and immune systems
- **Vibration:** Earthy and deep

LEGENDARY POWER

More than six thousand years ago, Malachite came from Egyptian copper mines in the Sinai that were sacred to the goddess Hathor (Venus). The huge Malachite columns in Istanbul's church of Hagia Sophia were recycled from an earlier temple of Diana at Ephesus.

Malachite was originally used as an amulet against enchantment and the evil eye. The ancients engraved the sun on the stone because they believed sunlight was antithetical to black magic, necromancers, and demons. Pliny tells us Malachite, a natural prophylactic against danger, benefited nursing mothers and protected children. Throughout the ancient and medieval worlds, the stone was used for healing the eyes. According to an ancient rhyme, "Opaque in hue, with th' emerald's vivid green [Malachite] charms the sight."

HEALING POWER

Malachite is a powerful conduit for transferring energy into the body and for absorbing environmental pollution, such as geopathic stress, electromagnetic smog, and radiation. Its reputation includes healing arthritis, possibly due to the minute particles of copper it contains, which are absorbed into the wearer's bloodstream. The Egyptians used Malachite as a paste to treat the eyes, cholera, and infected wounds. The copper carbonate hydroxide in Malachite has recently been found to have an antibacterial effect, inhibiting pathogens such as staphylococcus. This effect would have been reinforced by the Egyptian custom of mixing powdered Malachite with honey, a natural antibiotic.

Medieval lapidaries recommended Malachite for curing cramps and seizures and for easing childbirth. Crystal workers today use it to draw dis-ease from body and soul, and to assist psychosexual difficulties. On the physical level, it cleanses and regulates the body's organs. At the psychosomatic level, it dissolves the deeper causes of dis-ease. Malachite is best used under the guidance of an experienced crystal worker.

TRANSFORMATIONAL POWER

Malachite is a power stone for intense inner transformation and soul catharsis. This crystal is merciless in exposing personality imperfections, outgrown patterns, blockages, and ties that must be dissolved before you can evolve spiritually. It requires you to take responsibility for your thoughts, feelings, and actions. This makes it an excellent karmic and soul cleanser, activating your soul's purpose.

Malachite scours away the residue of traumas from past lifetimes or childhood and resets ancestral DNA. It then draws in spiritual energy to raise the frequency of your physical body. (Caution: Malachite is toxic in large quantities. Use polished stones, and wash your hands thoroughly after handling.)

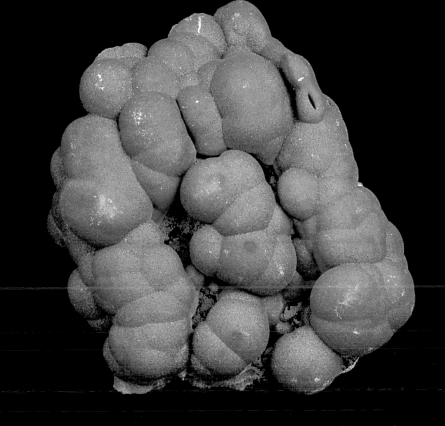

Meditate with Malachite, letting
your half-focused eyes follow
its contours. This journeying
or scrying stone takes you ever
deeper into yourself or the future.

Menalite

- **Chakra correspondences:** Earth star, base, sacral, past life
- **Physiological correspondences:** Breasts, hormonal production, endocrine and female reproductive systems
- **Vibration:** Earthy

LEGENDARY POWER

Holding the wise feminine and priestess power, Menalite connects you to the Earth Mother. This stone's Flint-like center provides stability during ritual work, especially rites of passage or fertility rituals. Excellent for shamanic journeying, it invites in power animals. Working with Menalite constructs a shamanic anchor that links your feet into the Earth and helps you feel at home on the planet.

Menalite reminds you that in ancient times, menstruation was a sacred process. Menstrual blood was offered to the goddess to ensure continued fertility and stabilize creation. The menstrual hut was sacred, a place of solitude and sisterhood where women dreamt their dreams. Divination and prophecy held sway. That sacredness has been lost, along with respect for the Crone, the female elder of the tribe whose wisdom was honored.

This stone assists in regaining respect and understanding of the sacred wisdom held in blood. Menalite guards and guides the soul as it incarnates, from conception through pregnancy to birth and on through the rites of passage that mark the stages of womanhood: child, maiden, mother, crone.

HEALING POWER

By solidifying the core energy field, Menalite assists during puberty and menopause by adjusting and rebalancing your subtle hormonal system, and provides psychological support in times of change. The stone energetically guards a mother and unborn child through pregnancy to birth, then encourages mother-child bonding and increased lactation. Hold Menalite during night sweats or hot flashes to draw out heat and moisture, calm the energy body, and promote restful sleep. At a psychological level, Menalite comforts women who have lost children or who are suffering from empty-nest syndrome.

TRANSFORMATIONAL POWER

This stone aids transformational work during transition stages of life: birth, puberty, menopause, and death. By removing fear, it lets you feel part of the power of creation and the endless cycles of life. It also aids in calling back and reintegrating fragments of your soul. Menalite helps you free yourself from family curses and past conditioning, removing their influence on you and breaking cycles of addiction or abuse. It assists in transforming dysfunctional families into harmonious units, although this work requires the guidance of a qualified therapist. If you have been affected by issues such as female circumcision, or if cultural attitudes about menstruation have made you feel unclean, Menalite reinstates your female power. With its assistance, you birth your true wise-woman self.

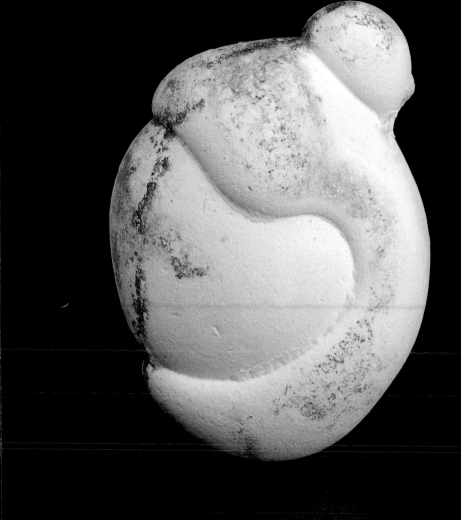

Put Menalite under your pillow to reconnect to the ancient feminine wisdom within the stone. Let it accompany you through the great transitions of life.

Merlinite

- **Chakra correspondences:** Past life, soma, third eye, higher heart (thymus)
- **Physiological correspondences:** Neurotransmitters; nervous, respiratory, and circulatory systems; etheric bodies; works mostly at a nonphysical level
- **Vibration:** High to very high (Mystic Merlinite)

LEGENDARY POWER

Containing eons of shamanic wisdom, Merlinite links into soul destiny and the Akashic Record. In Mesopotamia, the Record was known as the Tablets of Destinies. In Egypt, the god Thoth recorded actions, thoughts, and motives that were presented at the weighing of the heart ritual after death. The Jews had a "Book of Life," the Christians a Recording Angel, the Greeks the goddess Nemesis who ruled fate. In India, the *Akasha*, Sanskrit meaning "cosmic sky," was a nonphysical plane of existence where all human history was encoded.

The Record can be viewed as a hologram of everything that is and might be; our souls carry small pieces of the hologram. We play out the destinies we planned for ourselves in the space between lives, although this plan may be affected by accrued karma and outdated soul plans. By accessing the Akashic Record, we can see what we have been and what we might be, our potential futures depending on the choices we make now.

In science, the connectivity hypothesis suggests a subquantum energy field exists in which everything that happens is holographically—and permanently—recorded. Quantum physics also shows how future possibilities are encoded in this field. Merlinite facilitates connection to this cosmic memory field and to your soul's journey.

HEALING POWER

Crystal workers use Merlinite to balance mind, body, and spirit, and to bring masculine and feminine energies into equilibrium. It realigns neurotransmitters to accommodate expanded vibrational energy. Merlinite's greatest gift is karmic healing.

TRANSFORMATIONAL POWER

Merlinite helps you release the past and access the future. Placed on the past life chakras, it lets you see habitual patterns, past conditioning, and sources of karmic wounds. It helps you respond anew instead of with a conditioned reaction. Moments of great emotional trauma and soul dramas make the biggest impression on the Record. With the aid of a skilled past-life worker and Merlinite, you can reframe such scenes into a different outcome or discover the deeper meaning behind an apparently false scenario, as it is possible to tune into a historical event without actually having been there. By revealing why you choose the relationships you do, Merlinite attunes you to the various potential futures existing in each moment, each outcome stemming from a different choice. Mystic Merlinite takes you into ever-higher dimensions of your soul.

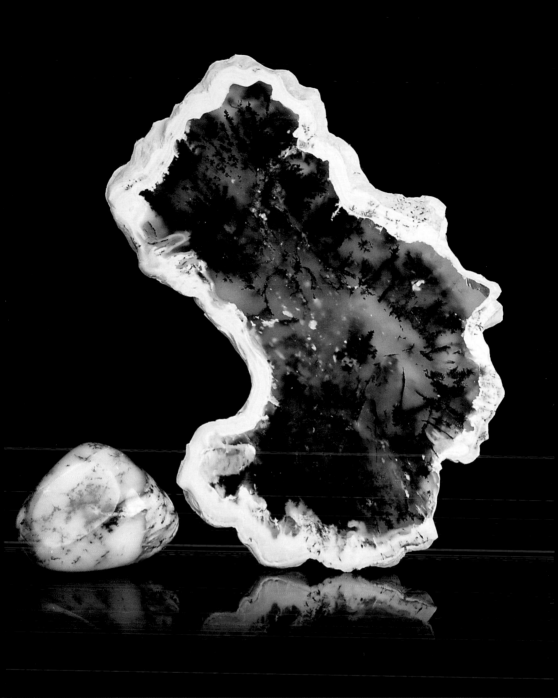

Place Merlinite over your third
eye to see the potential outcomes
of choices you have to make in
your present life.

Moldavite

- **Chakra correspondences:** All
- **Physiological correspondences:** Lightbody, underlying psychosomatic causes
- **Vibration:** High when genuine (artificially created Moldavite has no power and the characteristic "energy rush" of Moldavite is not present)

LEGENDARY POWER

Eleven million years ago, Moldavite burst onto Earth with enormous force as a giant meteor strike metamorphosed rock into a glass-like substance, fusing the power of the sky with that of Mother Earth. A metaphor for cosmic transformation, Moldavite was one of the highest vibration crystals for expanding consciousness, but it has now been surpassed. If you already work with high vibrations, you may have moved beyond Moldavite. However, its vibrations have recently been uplifted, and if you are new to crystals, it is a useful first step to higher-dimensional crystal working.

Many myths tell of a stone falling to Earth. In Eschenbach's *Parzival*, the Holy Grail was a green stone that fell from the sky, and many crystal authorities link Moldavite with the Grail. Another legend says that a green stone dropped from Satan's crown as he tumbled from heaven, a symbol of divine light falling to Earth. In the original myth, God's favorite angel was not evil, he was the light-bringer, as is Moldavite. Prized as a carrier of cosmic wisdom, it puts you in touch with higher guidance, planetary and star beings, ascended masters, and cosmic messengers.

More than twenty-five thousand years ago, the people of Eastern Europe used Moldavite as a talisman to enhance fertility and good fortune and fashioned tools from it. The stone is becoming rare.

HEALING POWER

Most people feel a rush of energy through their physical bodies when holding Moldavite. Rather than dealing with dis-ease itself, Moldavite focuses your attention on the cause. It helps to rectify underlying imbalances that create dis-ease and impede spiritual evolution. Grounding stones may be needed as Moldavite can cause dizziness.

If you are a star child who finds Earth's vibration heavy and inert, Moldavite adjusts your vibration to bring more cosmic energy down into your body, so you feel more at home at Earth while simultaneously transmuting Earth energy into cosmic light.

TRANSFORMATIONAL POWER

A crystal of karmic and soul transformation, Moldavite downloads information from the Akashic Record and instills cosmic consciousness. It takes you back into your past to reconnect to your previous wisdom and soul purpose, and into the future to access what you need for your soul's evolution. Then it lets you put that knowledge into practice in the present. (Note: if you are sensitive or unaccustomed to high-vibration crystals, wear or use Moldavite sparingly until an energetic adjustment is made.)

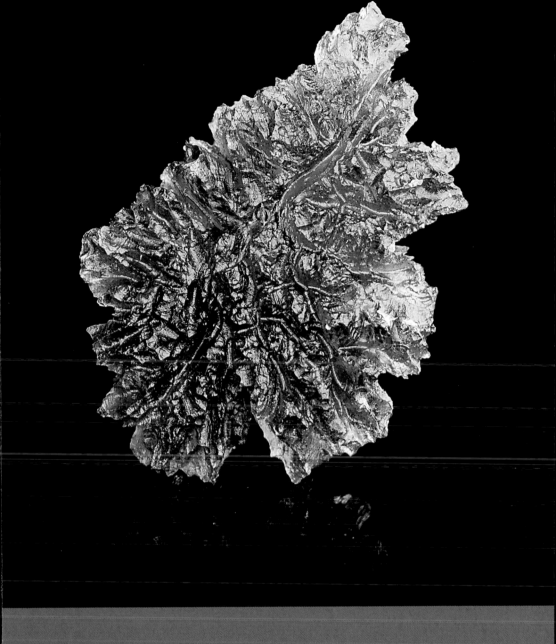

Meditate with Moldavite on your
third eye to connect to the highest
planes of consciousness and
become one with the cosmos.

Morganite
(Pink Beryl)

- **Chakra correspondences:** Heart, higher heart (thymus), heart seed, solar plexus

- **Physiological correspondences:** Nervous system, cells; psychosomatic conditions or emotional toxicity that affect eyes, heart, liver, lungs, stomach, throat, and cause seizures

- **Vibration:** High

LEGENDARY POWER

Morganite is a crystal of unconditional love and enormous forgiveness. Pink is the only color of Beryl not mentioned by Pliny, but this does not mean it was unknown as it is seen in Egyptian ritual jewelry. Beryl is a foundation stone of heaven in the Old and New Testaments. In an early Christian lapidary, Gregory the Great assigned crystals to nine orders of angels, Beryl being a stone of the Angelic Powers.

Although sharing the generic properties of Beryl, Morganite has its own unique vibration with a specific healing intention. It teaches the soul how to release feelings and experiences that have become toxic. These can block the heart and prevent the higher heart and heart seed chakras, which contain the temple of the inner self, from opening. Once the blocks have been released with the assistance of Morganite, your soul can reclaim that temple as its own sacred inner space.

HEALING POWER

Morganite works most effectively at the psychosomatic level of healing, but holds the emotional body stable while deep changes take place. Psychosomatic means illness aggravated or caused by an internal conflict or stress. Emotions, thoughts, and ingrained beliefs influence physical well-being, as do repressed feelings and unfulfilled emotional needs. Psychosomatic healing addresses issues that lie beneath an apparently physical disease. Simply having Morganite in the vicinity—especially when combined with Azeztulite (page 46)—brings these to the surface. Morganite also helps to dissolve subconscious resistance and fear of being healed. If you are comfortable with your pain and afraid to move forward, this crystal gently shows you that it is safe to step into well-being.

Crystal workers use Morganite to heal stress-related illnesses, to heal the heart, and aid lung conditions, such as asthma, emphysema, and TB. It may help to restructure and reenergize cells, ameliorate vertigo, and overcome impotence at a physical or emotional level.

TRANSFORMATIONAL POWER

Morganite helps you recognize the escape routes and evasive strategies you employ to avoid confronting core issues. By highlighting where closed-mindedness (a major cause of disease in Tibetan medicine) or egotism blocks your progress, it shows you the unfulfilled needs of your soul. With this powerful crystal, you can change a victim mentality into one of power and grace.

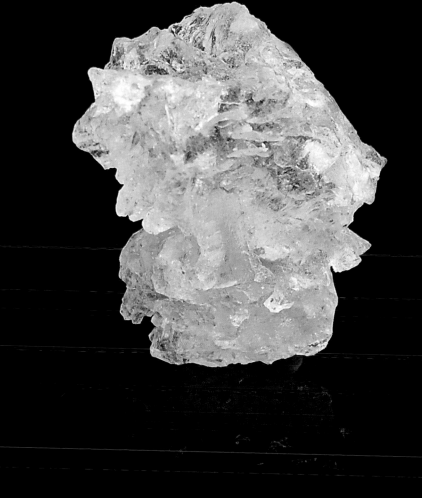

Place Morganite on your heart
chakra to gently bring repressed
feelings to the surface for
forgiveness and release, letting
your soul move forward with love.

Moss Agate

- **Chakra correspondences:** Earth, base, sacral, throat
- **Physiological correspondences:** Lymphatic, cellular, circulatory, reproductive and nervous systems, neurotransmitters, eyes, joints, heart
- **Vibration:** Earthy

LEGENDARY POWER

Moss Agate is the Mocha Stone mentioned in ancient lapidaries and was highly prized in the ancient world for its therapeutic and talismanic properties. As Moss Agate contains particles of iron, it was considered protective. The Persians believed it conferred eloquence of speech, in addition to the generic properties of Agate.

Under the doctrine of signatures (meaning a thing that resembles something else holds, through its energetic signature, the same properties and offers a remedy for the condition), Moss Agate is in sympathy with nature. It aids people affected by extreme weather allergies or environmental pollutants. Moss Agate has long been believed to be connected to agriculture and devas, nature spirits who live within the Earth and govern plant growth. The devas' united field of intelligence incorporates air, earth, water, and fire. They reside at the energetic boundary where consciousness births itself into matter, and they facilitate that process.

Using Moss Agate while a crop was sown transferred fertility to the plants, ensuring a good yield. As the *Lithica* tells us, "If the same be tied to the horns of thine oxen when ploughing, or about the ploughman's sturdy arm, wheat-crowned Ceres shall descend from heaven with full lap upon thy furrows." Traditionally a "wet" stone, Moss Agate brought rain and ensured the right amount fell for crops to flourish.

HEALING POWER

Early midwives used Moss Agate in birthing work to reduce pain and encourage a safe delivery. In Chinese medicine, Moss Agate has long been employed to dispel confusion, and crystal workers use it to stabilize and strengthen the mind. Early medicine prescribed Moss Agate for the eyes. Physicians ground up medicinal powders on palettes made from Moss Agate, which transferred infinitesimal amounts of magnesium, manganese, and iron from the stone to the potion. Magnesium is necessary for enzyme functioning, energy transfer, healthy bones, and the proper working of muscles, nerves, and tissue. An anti-inflammatory, Moss Agate is used today to energetically heal the lymphatic system and dehydration, to heal skin and fungal infections, and to realign neurotransmitters.

TRANSFORMATIONAL POWER

A stone of new beginnings, Moss Agate helps you birth new projects and attract abundance. Its dual action assists people who are overly caught up in their feelings to be more objective, and lets those with overly intellectual minds get in touch with their feelings. (See Agate, page 20.)

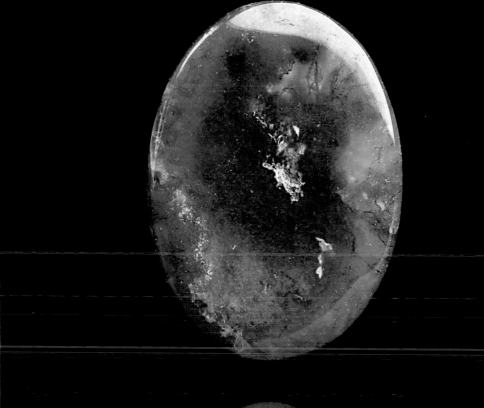

Meditate with Moss Agate to
reveal the core cause of a problem
and gain the persistence required
to overcome the situation.

Natrolite and Scolecite

- **Chakra correspondences:** Opens and aligns all chakras including highest crown
- **Physiological correspondences:** Etheric bodies, neurotransmitters, and nervous, muscular, and lymphatic systems
- **Vibration:** High to exceptionally high

LEGENDARY POWER

These stones look similar, but Scolecite is an energetically stepped-down version of Natrolite. In its pure white form, Natrolite, a sodium silicate, is virtually pure light. It brings about a profound shift in metaphysical and spiritual awareness, attuning you to the wisdom of universal mind and channeling light into your body.

Scolecite is a calcium silicate; its earthier vibration is suitable for beginners and for people with particularly sensitive energy fields. Check which crystal is most appropriate for you by placing Scolecite in your hand for a few moments and asking that the energies harmonize. If Scolecite feels comfortable, change to Natrolite. If Natrolite feels too strong, return to Scolecite and try Natrolite again after a few weeks. One of the stones will be more suitable according to how your physical realignment to the vibrational shift is progressing.

Using the two crystals in tandem creates a vibrational ladder that you can ascend to reach multidimensions, so that it becomes possible to live with complete awareness in several dimensions at once. This should only be attempted by experienced high-vibration crystal workers who have purified their physical energy to the most refined state possible. Otherwise, begin working with Scolecite and move to Natrolite when the necessary energetic cleansing and shifts have occurred.

To anchor the new energies firmly into your body and to assist assimilation, place a Smoky Elestial Quartz at your feet and Natrolite or Scolecite above your head. Scolecite digs out the last residues of outmoded patterns or attachments released by other stones from the aura.

HEALING POWER

Natrolite realigns the subtle bodies and reattunes the nervous system and neurotransmitters after an influx of expanded consciousness. For disturbances of the body's nervous and muscular systems, such as muscular sclerosis, place Scolecite on the back and Natrolite on the front of your chakras. Put whichever crystal feels most appropriate over the thymus and head, and a grounding stone such as Hematite or Smoky Elestial at your feet. This layout may also rectify fluid or meridian imbalances. Grid this combination around your bed if too strong a vibrational influx causes insomnia.

TRANSFORMATIONAL POWER

The Natrolite-Scolecite combination transforms your physical body into a vehicle for the lightbody and expanded consciousness. If you find it difficult to function on the Earth due to your sensitivity to vibrational change, this realignment enables you to live comfortably within your physical body with an embodied spiritual self.

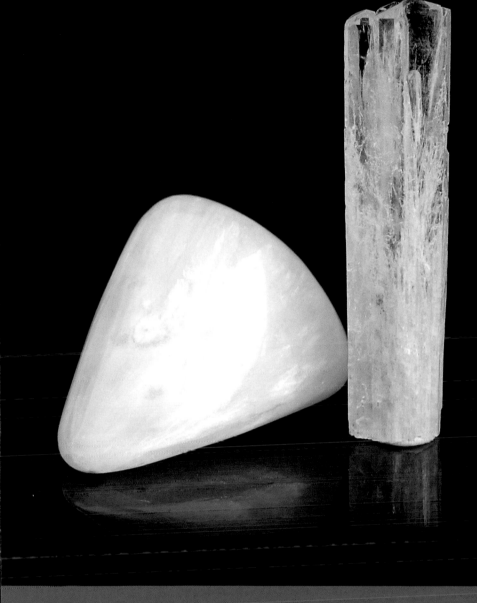

Use Scolecite and Natrolite in combination on the chakras to realign the energy bodies to higher vibrations and infuse your core being with inner peace.

Nirvana Quartz™

- **Chakra correspondences:** Soul star, stellar gateway, and beyond
- **Physiological correspondences:** Subtle biomagnetic fields, energy meridians, the lightbody
- **Vibration:** Exceptionally high

LEGENDARY POWER

Nirvana is one of the highest vibration Quartzes yet discovered. A crystal of spiritual alchemy, it attunes the flame of pure consciousness to the soul star chakra so that the light of expansion and enlightenment flows through the body and into the Earth.

The ancient Greek poet Orpheus tells us that Quartz is "the translucent image of the Eternal Light." Pliny attributes the formation of Quartz to the intense freezing of ice, and Claudianus called it "ice hardened into stone, which no frost could congeal nor dog-star [Sirius] dry up." Nirvana Quartz's scrunched and crumpled appearance makes it clear how such a belief came about. It looks exactly like compressed ice—appropriate given that Nirvana Quartz was born out of retreating glaciers high in the Himalayas and has a metaphysical connection to Sirius, one of the brightest stars.

Nirvana Quartz exists at the energetic interface between matter and consciousness, mind and body. Tibetan Buddhists prize it for deepening meditation. Being in the presence of Nirvana Quartz reveals that it is a true crystal of enlightenment and reminds us

The whole process of life is characterized as constant flux. Life is not static, but dynamic, and all moments of existence are intermediate states, even between two different states in the process of transformation. To recognize the changeable nature of the whole empirical world means to see its deceptive insubstantiality. Then there opens up the path to the unchangeable.
—Buddhist Sutra

HEALING POWER

Although found to be effective against chilblains, Nirvana Quartz works mostly beyond the physical level to create an enlightened heart, mind, and soul. Acting as an energetic bridge between a healer and a distant recipient, it assists a surrogate who is standing in for someone who needs soul retrieval or entity disconnection. However, this work requires an experienced healer. Nirvana Quartz may instigate a healing catharsis as the physical and subtle bodies are purified and karma released. Place Smoky Elestial Quartz at your feet to facilitate transmutation of energies set free by the process of spiritual alchemy.

TRANSFORMATIONAL POWER

With Nirvana Quartz, you become aware that you are a spiritual being on a human journey and your task is to bring divine light into the world to shift the perceptions of consensual reality into spiritual truth. (Note: Nirvana Quartz is often sold as Ice or Growth Interference Quartz, although there are subtle energetic differences between the different crystals.)

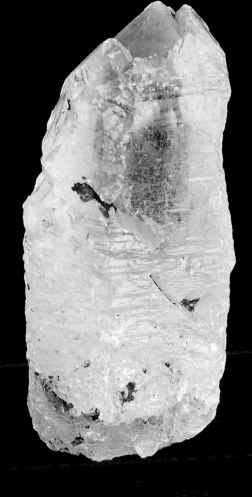

Meditate with Nirvana Quartz
to induce a bliss-like state of
unconditional love combined with
pure mind in which the divine
infuses the physical realm.

Novaculite

- **Chakra correspondences:** Crown, soul star, stellar gateway; removes cords from and realigns all chakras
- **Physiological correspondences:** Cellular structures, skin, etheric body
- **Vibration:** Earthy and extremely high

LEGENDARY POWER

Novaculite is similar to Flint and shares that stone's properties, including the ability to open portals to other worlds. For more than three thousand years, the ancient peoples of America created tools and decorative jewelry from this microcrystalline Quartz.

A useful adjunct to shamanic journeying, Novaculite hones your soul. It scours away all that is outworn and outgrown, especially cords that subtly bind you to the past. Having freed and realigned the chakras, it pulls spiritual energy down into your body. Novaculite harmonizes well with Nuummite to remove the effects of ancient sorcery and present-life curses, but it is best used by a qualified crystal worker.

HEALING POWER

Novaculite's very fine vibration aids multidimensional and environmental healing. Its focused beam of intense light rejigs the etheric blueprint so the physical body can come into a new alignment. Working mainly at the level of psyche and soul, Novaculite adjusts cellular memory and restructures genetic codes. At a psychological level, it reveals the reasons behind obsessive-compulsive disorders and balances bipolar swings. Washing with Novaculite-infused water is thought to maintain the elasticity of healthy skin and remove warts. Gridding Novaculite repairs and reenergizes the Earth's etheric matrix, restoring the flow of electromagnetic currents.

TRANSFORMATIONAL POWER

Novaculite means "razor," and this stone was traditionally used to sharpen tools; however, modern crystal workers use it to hone the soul. Inappropriate connections to the past can be detrimental to your physical energy and soul growth. If you are bound to another soul through past-life experiences, contracts, agreements, previous vows and promises, or a present-life interaction that has run its course, Novaculite lets you cut the cords between you. It reframes contracts into a more appropriate agenda or none at all. Particularly useful for higher-chakra cord-cutting, Novaculite sets you free to be who you are meant to be in the here and now. The stone teaches you to set appropriate boundaries: flexible and caring, yet resistant to energetic invasion or abuse.

No matter how traumatic a situation you may have endured, Novaculite identifies the gift in the experience. It helps you look to the stars and contact angelic guidance.

This stone smoothes the rough edges of a discordant personality and instills a quietly confident approach to life. If you tend to dwell on problems, Novaculite teaches you to give attention to solutions. (Caution: Novaculite shards can be extremely sharp.)

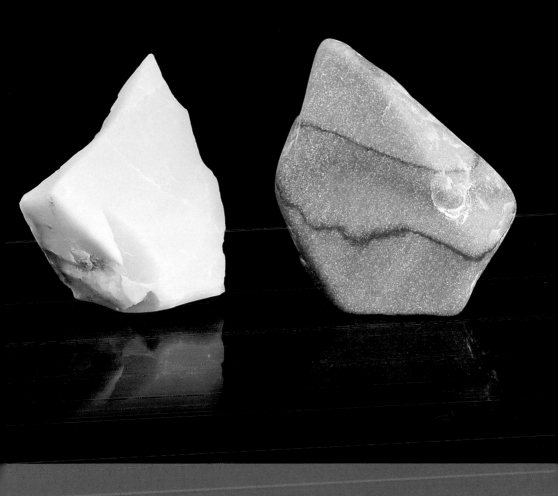

Sweep Novaculite away from the physical body to cut through subtle energetic ties that bind you to the past and seal where they've been.

Nuummite

- **Chakra correspondences:** Earth star, base, past life, soma; activates and integrates all chakras
- **Physiological correspondences:** Eyes, limbic brain, kidneys, cellular structures, reproductive and nervous systems, triple burner meridian, insulin regulation, subtle auric bodies
- **Vibration:** Earthy and high

LEGENDARY POWER

Nuummite carries the power of the void, which holds potent magic to be used with respect and right intention. In ancient creation myths, matter is born out of the void, formless space that existed before the material world. The apocryphal Wisdom of Solomon tells us it was the spirit of Wisdom (Sophia, eternal mind or consciousness) who "fashioned all things," suggesting that consciousness brought the world into being. It is Wisdom who "knows the things of old, and infers the things to come."

Created three billion years ago, Nuummite is the oldest mineral on the planet. It connects directly into the power of the void and its endless possibilities for creation and regeneration. Nuummite teaches you to value the dark places where all things compost and arise anew.

Traditionally the sorcerer's stone, Nuummite's iridescent surface sends out magical vibes that connect to the metaphysical world. It helps you journey safely through the realms of the subconscious and universal mind to inner awareness. Conveying stealth and cunning, Nuummite shields the aura. It turns back curses and releases the soul from karmic entanglements, mental imprints, and psychic manipulation.

HEALING POWER

Nuummite heals the etheric blueprint, cutting out karmic, emotional, or mental dis-ease that may manifest psychosomatically. By aligning the subtle and physical bodies, it removes energetic implants and heals auric weakness. Nuummite can be used by experienced crystal workers for psychic surgery on energy blockages and karmic debris.

Nuummite ameliorates mental causes of insomnia and protects the soul during sleep. By energetically regenerating the brain's limbic system and its cellular structures, and by recalibrating the subtle nervous system and neural pathways, it may aid Parkinson's and other degenerative dis-eases. Placed on the back of the neck, it may clear tension headaches; over the pancreas, it may regulate the flow of insulin; on the triple burner meridian, it balances energy and heat flow in the body.

TRANSFORMATIONAL POWER

If you have misused your power in this or another life, Nuummite teaches right use of power, making you aware that karma is created from every thought, word, and deed. Nuummite cuts to your core and creates you anew, teaching you to honor the darkness that contains your spiritual light. It brings you to a point of balance where light and darkness harmonize and complement each other. It reminds you to pay your dues and do only what is needful. In this way, true spiritual equilibrium is maintained.

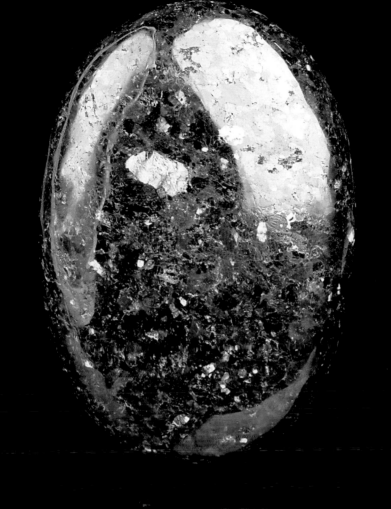

Meditate with Nuummite to
recognize debts from the past and
cut away all that is outgrown or
manipulative.

Obsidian

- **Chakra correspondences:** Earth star, base, sacral
- **Physiological correspondences:** Detoxification, digestive and circulation systems, joints, prostate
- **Vibration:** Earthy to medium, depending on color and type

LEGENDARY POWER

This stone has long been regarded as a magical portal through time and space. Theophrastus tells us the ancient Greeks gazed into scrying mirrors made from polished Obsidian, and Obsidian crystal balls have been used for thousands of years.

Obsidian is a shamanic tool for removing blockages and debris from the past. It blocks psychic attack or harmful intentions by providing a shield for the aura. Gentle Apache Tears are the most suitable Obsidian to carry for this purpose. Rainbow Obsidian cuts through energetic cords that bind two souls together inappropriately. With this stone's assistance, you can free yourself to love again.

HEALING POWER

Best used under the supervision of a qualified crystal healer, Obsidian works rapidly. It may bring on a healing challenge or provoke an emotional catharsis, and it reveals the reasons behind a dis-ease. Mahogany, Snowflake, Apache Tear, and Blue Obsidians work at a gentler pace than Black. Merciless in exposing character traits that require transformation, Obsidian encourages deep soul healing. It clears outdated mental constructs and thought forms, highlighting with absolute clarity what must change. Place Obsidian in a healing room to facilitate rapid release of core issues and absorb the negative energies released.

At a physical level, Obsidian draws off negativity, assisting the body's structures to energetically detoxify, soften, and realign. It aids past-life healing where unpleasant facts or deep trauma need to be faced and transformed.

TRANSFORMATIONAL POWER

If you have lost your power, Obsidian helps you address the issue and re-empower yourself. It lets you look in the mirror of your inner being, going deep into the subconscious, facing what has to be faced, integrating your shadow, and transmuting the negativity of lifetimes to free your soul. With the Black variety you can explore and reframe the ancestral line. This is a stone of deep integrity that brings you back to your spiritual path.

Spider Web Obsidian helps you recognize the patterns that hold you in the past and the controls you put in place. It shows how you manipulated yourself and others—the web you wove in order to survive. This stone pulls no punches, but is gentler than some Obsidians. With its assistance, you can bring your innermost designs to the surface and consciously create a web of light that supports what you most desire. It reveals the beauty you hold in the recesses of your soul.

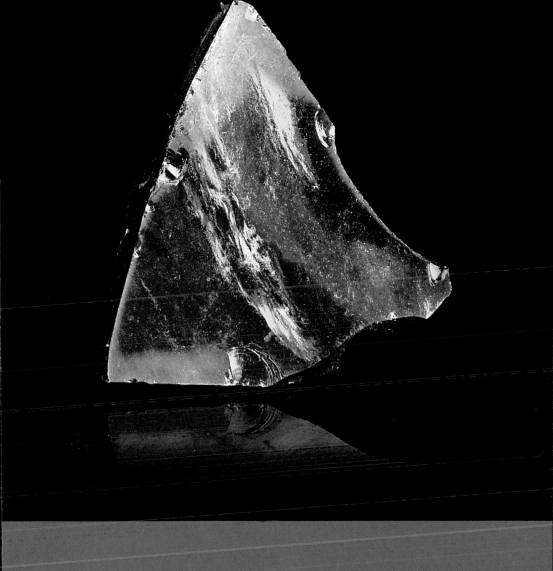

Place Obsidian at your feet.
Visualize cords passing from each
foot, going through the earth star,
entwining deep into the Earth,
anchoring you during turmoil.

Opal

- **Chakra correspondences:** Third eye, heart
- **Physiological correspondences:** Blood, kidneys, pancreas, reproductive organs, eyes, neurotransmitters, hair, nails, abdomen, intestines, triple burner meridian, immune system
- **Vibration:** Earthy to high, depending on type

LEGENDARY POWER

Opal symbolizes hope, innocence, and purity. The name comes from the Sanskrit word *upala* meaning "precious," and Pliny opines, "some by their refulgent splendor rival the colors of the painters." Brittle due to high water content, it fractures easily, but paradoxically, its amorphous structure allows vibrations to pass rapidly through the crystal.

Opal's legendary powers center around mysterious fatalities, and it has an almost physical, kinesthetic power of influence. King Alfonso XII of Spain gave his wife an Opal ring on their wedding day. She died soon after, so he presented it to his sister, who died a few days later. His sister-in-law lasted three months. He wore it himself but soon died, whereupon the crystal was hung on the statute of the Virgin of Almudena. The deaths ceased.

In Greco-Roman times, Opal was associated with Hermes/Mercury, who conveyed the souls of the dead to the underworld. Opal saw into these realms; it focused thought and restored memory. Opal lets you travel unseen through the shamanic otherworld or into dangerous places as it confers invisibility on the wearer and protects against the evil eye. An Elizabethan lapidary says Opal:

> *keepeth and saveth his eyen [eyes] that beareth it, cleare and sharpe and without griefe, and dimmeth other men's eyes . . . and smiteth them with a manner blindness . . .*
> *Therefore it is said that it is the most sure patron of thieves.*

Holding an Opal in the left hand and gazing into its depths allegedly attracted all you desired. Opal illustrates that we create our own "good" or "bad" fortune with our beliefs and intentions. The crystal helps you be pure in heart and strengthens your power of thought.

HEALING POWER

Traditionally used for healing the eyes, Opal's high silica content may benefit hair, nails, and skin. Modern crystal workers use Opal to purify the blood, ease PMS, and energetically stabilize neurotransmitter disturbances, such as Parkinson's.

TRANSFORMATIONAL POWER

Opal picks up thoughts and feelings and reflects them back to their source so their effect might be better understood. It teaches that what you put out returns to you. Oregon Opal, in particular, helps you identify untruths and deceptions—from yourself or others—that undermine your well-being. It helps you transform your life by standing in truth. (Note: Porous Opal should not be immersed in water. Oil restores luster to cabochon-cut stones.)

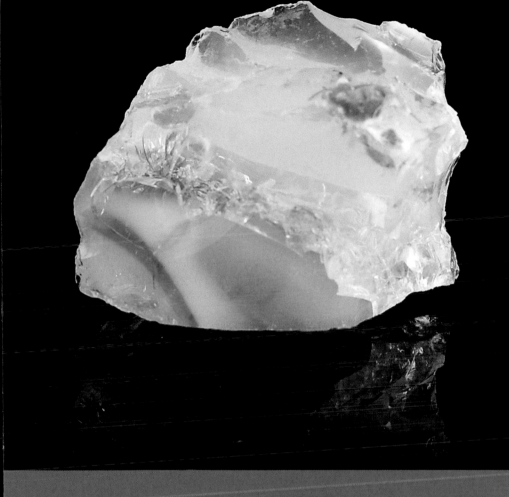

Hold your Opal, focus your
attention into the crystal,
and visualize what you wish to
manifest. It will come into being.

Orange Kyanite

- **Chakra correspondences:** Earth star, base, sacral; energizes and aligns all chakras
- **Physiological correspondences:** Brain, especially the cerebellum, throat, adrenal glands, urogenital system, blood pressure, motor function
- **Vibration:** High

LEGENDARY POWER

Orange Kyanite is an exciting find from Tanzania that looks like crystallized sunshine and fizzes with energy. It potentizes your personal creative power and manifestation abilities. The color comes from manganese; the golden "scales" are mica, which refines and radiates high-frequency energy. This vibrant form of Kyanite grounds ideas in the everyday world. All Kyanites are excellent amplifiers and transmitters of energy, but Orange reaches a very high vibration indeed, helping you delve deeply into your psyche to find and release causal connections behind karmic or creative blockages.

Orange Kyanite also lets you look within to find the roots of your passion and pleasure. It energizes the sacral chakra, the center of procreation and acceptance of yourself as a sexual being, bringing success to all creative endeavors. If the sacral chakra is blocked, low self-esteem and a sense of inferiority result, which may be hidden behind cruelty, pomposity, jealousy, or general sluggishness. Infertility or inability to put plans into action indicates that hooks from other people, especially from sexual encounters, may be blocking the sacral chakra. Orange Kyanite energetically detaches these and heals the site.

Orange Kyanite opens, cleanses, and infuses all the chakras with light. It opens psychic channels, facilitates higher attunement, and brings spiritual energy into manifestation. Negativity cannot stick to Kyanite. It dispels karmic blockages that hold you back, especially those arising from past-life sexual experiences or beliefs.

Kyanite is sometimes called *disthene*, meaning "twice," because it has positive and negative electrical polarity. This stone activates the positive dragon (or kundalini) energy within the universe.

HEALING POWER

Apply Orange Kyanite to the meridians and organs of the belly to energetically dissolve underlying dis-ease, the effects of which may include PMS, muscle cramps, impotence, infertility, allergies, diabetes, liver or intestinal dysfunction, irritable bowel, chronic back pain, and urinary infections. This stone also helps reveal the hidden causes of addictions and eating disorders, reprogramming the brain to have a more functional approach to the body.

TRANSFORMATIONAL POWER

With the assistance of Orange Kyanite, you operate from a higher level of creativity because you are in touch with the manifestation forces of the universe. You program your lightbody to operate in the everyday world with minimum effort and maximum effect. You literally create a new world.

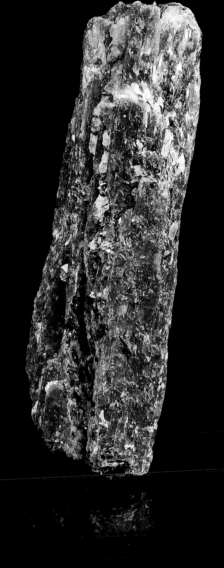

Place Orange Kyanite over the
sacral chakra five minutes a day
to become an assertive, creative,
confident person who takes
pleasure in life and love.

Paraiba Tourmaline

- **Chakra correspondences:** Stellar gateway, heart seed, heart, higher heart (thymus), third eye; aligns all chakras and seals the aura
- **Physiological correspondences:** Stomach, throat, eyes, jaw, thyroid gland, filtration organs, and metabolic, immune, and hormonal systems
- **Vibration:** Very high

LEGENDARY POWER

Radiant Paraiba Tourmaline polarizes light and shines it into the recesses of your heart and soul, lighting up your inner being. Generic Tourmaline's properties are unique in the mineral kingdom; most were only identified in the eighteenth century, and many were not accepted at that time. The ensuing scientific argument was finally settled by experiments, illustrating how truth must be tested against existing beliefs and, if appropriate, those beliefs must be amended.

Some of Tourmaline's qualities seem almost magical. If, for instance, two slices of Tourmaline are laid on top of each other with their axes parallel, they appear transparent when viewed from one direction, but opaque when seen from another. Tourmaline also has double refraction and exhibits remarkable electrical activity when heated or excited by friction. If the crystal is broken, the ends act like the polarities of a magnet.

Tourmaline's dichroism explains why Paraiba may appear green or purple when viewed from different angles. This stone is sought after for its vibrant, copper-based blue-green color. Many faceted Paraibas have been heat-treated to bring out the intense color, a magical feat of crystal alchemy.

HEALING POWER

Paraiba works mostly at the emotional and spiritual levels, encouraging forgiveness and releasing bitterness in the heart. Physically, it acts as an energetic tonic and may assist filtration. Crystal workers use it to calm sore throats and swollen glands, alleviate hay fever, and stimulate the thyroid. Green Tourmalines are traditionally used to heal the eyes and to stimulate the body's cleansing and elimination systems. Paraiba is excellent for removing pollutants from the subtle energy bodies.

TRANSFORMATIONAL POWER

Paraiba works its magical transformations on several levels. A stone of compassionate being, it stimulates the radiant heart, opening the heart seed chakra and bringing unconditional love into the Earth plane. It teaches you how to love yourself and others from the soul's perspective. Stimulating spiritual evolution by opening the stellar gateway, it identifies where you have strayed from your truth, bringing you back to the path of awareness and facilitating expression of your true feelings. If outdated, ingrained beliefs, karmic wounds, or mental constructs are blocking the way, Paraiba gently dissolves them and helps you forgive yourself and others.

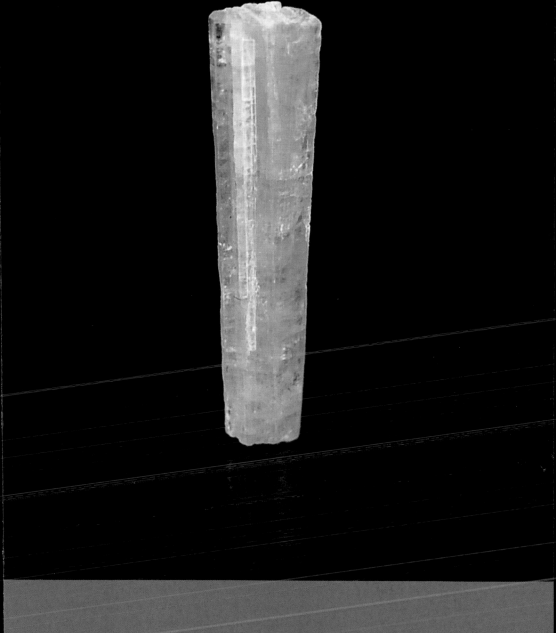

Place Paraiba Tourmaline over the past life chakra for a few minutes each day to bring unfinished business to its natural conclusion.

Peridot (Chrysolite)

- **Chakra correspondences:** Heart, solar plexus
- **Physiological correspondences:** Eyes, heart, thymus, lungs, skin, spleen, gallbladder, intestines, digestive system, metabolic processes
- **Vibration:** Earthy to high

LEGENDARY POWER

In the eighth century, the Archbishop of Mainz called Peridot one of the twelve Apostolic gems ensuring "true spiritual preaching accompanied by miracles." The thirteenth-century *Book of Wings* tells us that a talisman of Peridot carved with a vulture "constrains demons and the wind." It forced the demons to cease their importuning and put them under the wearer's control—a tradition dating from Greco-Roman times and earlier.

According to Pliny, in ancient Rome, Peridot was preferred above any other stone. Allegedly, it was the largest gemstone and, being soft, could be shaped with an iron file. Although it was discovered before Pliny's time, he passed on information collected over millennia. He tells us that piratical Troglodytes, or cave dwellers, exhausted from storms and hunger, came ashore on an Arabian island. While digging for roots, they unearthed a Peridot. Since then, the stone has been highly regarded for its power of manifestation. Almost certainly one of the stones from the Breastplate of the High Priest and a foundation for the New Jerusalem, Peridot is a stone for Archangel Raphael and rules the realm of Angelic Virtues.

HEALING POWER

The magician Agrippa tells us that in German High Magic, a Peridot held to the sun "shines forth a golden star," comforting the respiratory system and healing asthma. Peridot had a reputation for healing eye diseases. Traditionally used to strengthen contractions, it promoted a painless birth. Peridot is a powerful energetic cleanser on all levels. Modern crystal workers use it to energetically balance the swings of bipolar disorder and to overcome hypochondria; it may also strengthen and detox blood-rich organs.

TRANSFORMATIONAL POWER

Agrippa suggests that a Peridot bound to the left arm drives away "idle imaginations and melancholy fears, putting away foolishness." It has long been used to overcome psychiatric disturbances and cut psychological bonds to achieve mental clarity. It detaches your mind from external influences and clears negative thought patterns, teaching you how to find your inner guidance and access the wisdom of the higher mind. If you tend to blame others, Peridot insists you take responsibility for yourself. If you suffer from spite, jealousy, or resentment, meditating with Peridot instills confidence in your own abilities and teaches you to be content with your lot. A crystal of forgiveness and insight, it also helps you admit mistakes and overcome psychological lethargy. If you have lost your sense of direction, wearing Peridot reconnects you to your destiny.

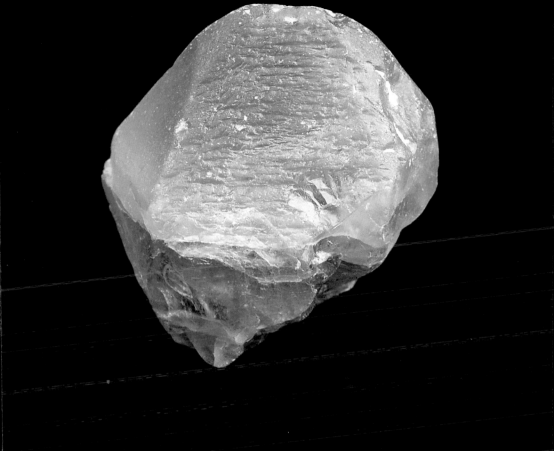

Draw a five-pointed star.
Place Peridots on each point and
a picture of what you wish to manifest
in the center. Concentrate, then
withdraw attention.

Petalite

- **Chakra correspondences:** Soul star, stellar gateway, crown, soma, third eye
- **Physiological correspondences:** Subtle bodies, respiratory, cellular memory, triple burner meridian, eyes, intestines, metabolic and endocrine systems
- **Vibration:** Exceptionally high

LEGENDARY POWER

Walt Whitman described cosmic consciousness as "ineffable light, light rare, untellable, light beyond all signs, descriptions and languages," a definition that fits Petalite. With this ethereal crystal, you move beyond the personal "I" of human perception and merge with all *knowing*. Holding it creates a safe space in which to open higher awareness and obtain profound metaphysical insights. Often known as "the Angel stone," Petalite connects you with the angelic realm and ascended masters.

By opening the third eye and linking the throat and crown chakras, Petalite lets you share your enhanced spiritual insight and ultimate truth. Its powerful karmic clearing effect purifies all the subtle bodies; it is extremely effective as crystal-infused water rubbed over the past life and soma chakras. Petalite promotes ancestral and family healing—its effects go back through generations to a time before the dysfunction was created. It then takes the new energy into the future, so a pristine functional pattern can be set in place.

If you need to cut ties with your family or release previous relationships to clear karma and outgrown expectations so that unconditional love and forgiveness can flow in, hold pink Petalite while you visualize the ties being dissolved. Call in your higher self and the other person's to explain why you are cutting these ties. Petalite assures you the process will not cut off unconditional soul love between you; your higher self ensures the cutting is effected at higher frequencies as well as that of the Earth plane. Both souls can then go forward, free to be as they are meant to be.

HEALING POWER

Petalite works beyond the physical level to harmonize the metaphysical activity of the pineal and pituitary glands. It aligns the metabolic system to higher frequencies, adjusts cellular memory, and purifies the subtle bodies.

For people with cancer or AIDS, Petalite facilitates understanding the spiritual reasons for taking on dis-ease. It energetically activates cell membranes to manifest wellness, and gently dissolves resistance to transition. Crystal healers use it to heal eyes, lungs, muscles, and intestines. Because it contains lithium, Petalite energetically ameliorates depression. This powerful emotional healer gently dissolves feelings of abandonment and alienation, and brings you home to your true soul family.

TRANSFORMATIONAL POWER

By connecting you to cosmic consciousness, Petalite makes you aware of the breadth of your soul and of higher realities. This gentle crystal rapidly accelerates your spiritual evolution.

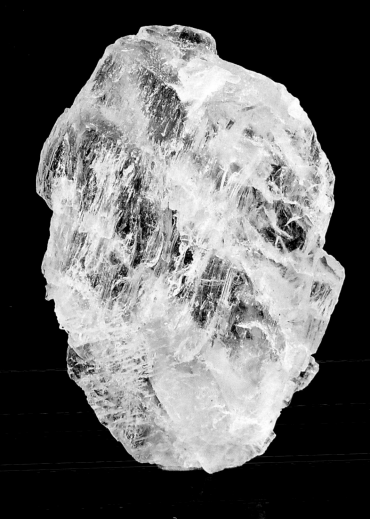

Meditating with Petalite
brings divine light and cosmic
consciousness into the physical
plane, speeding up the evolution of
humanity and the Earth itself.

Petrified Wood

- **Chakra correspondences:** Earth star, base, sacral, solar plexus, higher heart (thymus)
- **Physiological correspondences:** Immune system, joints, muscles, bones, feet, motility, back, nervous system, lungs, the aging process, disintegration, calcification, sleep patterns, twelve-strand DNA
- **Vibration:** Earthy; grounds high-vibration stones

LEGENDARY POWER

Petrified forests were places of enchantment, where witches and gods had magically transformed wood into stone. Part of the cosmic battle between good and evil, fossilized trees were believed in India to be the bones of a demon slain by Lord Vishnu. In a Dutch folktale, millions of good fairies came from the sun to take up residence in the Earth and metamorphosed into trees. These trees had the power to heal, but were cut down and driven into the soil to stabilize the land.

Legends abound about the healing properties of trees. Petrified Wood helps you explore previous incarnations—read each ring as a lifetime.

HEALING POWER

Petrified Wood creates core stability and adjusts energetic flow to optimum. Crystal workers use it when locomotion—or life—is a challenge. Placed over the higher heart (thymus) chakra it energetically opens up the lungs, increases oxygen intake, and brings new energy into the subtle and physical bodies, assisting chronic fatigue syndrome, convalescence, and exhaustion. Holding it provides emotional comfort during a healing challenge or when a burden seems too much to bear. If DNA potential is blocked by ancestral genetic memory, Petrified Wood unlocks the molecular gates that held the cell captive.

TRANSFORMATIONAL POWER

Truly an allegory for spiritual alchemy, Petrified Wood began as a living tree, which then lay in mineral-rich water. If the water was infused with volcanic ash, the molecules of wood were replaced with shining silica so that no trace of organic material remained. The rings and knots remained visible and mineral impurities created beautiful colors. Polishing reveals these colors, just as incarnation polishes the soul; thus, Petrified Wood represents the strength and beauty of your soul.

This crystal provides support during the trials and tribulations of spiritual evolution, showing you the soul gifts that challenges offer. It lets you peel back the layers encasing your core being, releasing all that no longer serves you while retaining what does. By helping you feel at home on the Earth, it reminds you that you are more than spirit trapped within the material world and that one day you'll rise again to take on another form. In the meantime, give service to your earthly home. This crystal shows how to walk upon the Earth with grace, honoring the wisdom of the ages.

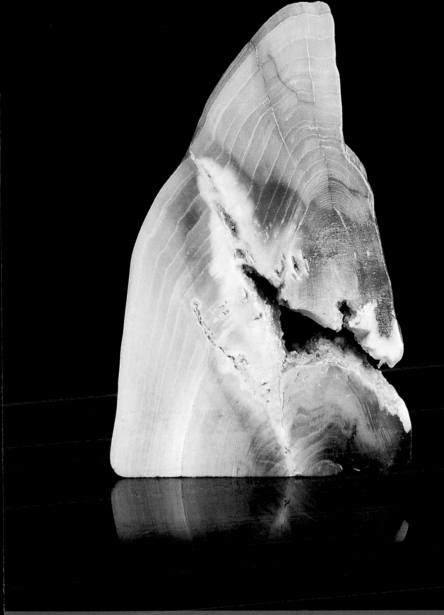

Holding Petrified Wood keeps
your feet firmly on the ground
while you explore multidimensions
of reality and transforms you into a
soul being of light.

Phenacite in Red Feldspar

- **Chakra correspondences:** Opens, heals, and activates all chakras to a high level
- **Physiological correspondences:** Etheric blueprint, muscles
- **Vibration:** Earthy and exceedingly high

LEGENDARY POWER

Phenacite in Red Feldspar is an exciting stone with enormous power to facilitate life-changing shifts and open endless possibilities. This rare and powerful synergistic combination unites the high vibrations and profound spiritual insight of Phenacite with the grounded vibrations of Red Feldspar to anchor information into the material world. It steps down the highest of frequencies to a level accessible to Earth, while protecting the pure essence of the transmission. The effect is greater than individual stones but, if the combination isn't available, two individual stones can work together. Choose a Phenacite that you feel has the strongest vibration, as crystals from various locations interact differently according to your own level of attunement.

Phenacite (on the left in this photo) was known as "the deceiver," as it was often mistaken for Diamond. Few were found outside Russia before the nineteenth century, when Phenacites from a Colorado find were cut into brilliant gemstones. Its value has risen dramatically in the last few decades as its exceedingly high vibration has been recognized.

Phenacite crystals are doubly refractive—they help you see into the heart of a matter and bring information from the highest reaches of consciousness into the material world. Connecting to ascended masters and the Akashic Record, the crystal is particularly useful for dream work; the combination stone unravels the deeper meaning of a prophetic dream.

Earthy Red Feldspar works on the physical and subtle bodies to release the ingrained patterns of the past held within the etheric blueprint. It prepares the physical body for a more dynamic and active way of being.

HEALING POWER

This stone works mainly at the energetic level to heal the etheric blueprint, effecting multidimensional cellular healing and settling that within the physical body through enhanced neural transmission. Placed on the back of the neck, the combination enhances memory and may benefit muscular problems.

TRANSFORMATIONAL POWER

If you've been hesitant to begin your spiritual path, this combination gets you moving—but it also knows about right timing. It instigates action that is perfectly attuned to your highest good. I nicknamed it "Kick Ass" because it does exactly that. If something is stuck in your life, this combination ejects unwanted visitors (physical or discarnate) and rapidly dissolves blockages, triggering your soul purpose and drastically changing your reality. It teaches that spiritual evolution is a joyful process.

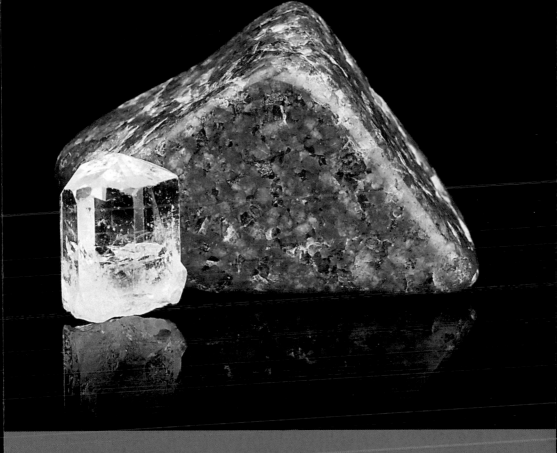

This combination accelerates your consciousness to lift off into the lightness of being. Obstacles in your life will melt away.

Poppy Jasper

- **Chakra correspondences:** Earth star, base, sacral, solar plexus; aligns all chakras and strengthens the aura
- **Physiological correspondences:** Circulation, digestion, sexual function, reproductive organs, liver, bile ducts, mineral assimilation
- **Vibration:** Earthy

LEGENDARY POWER

Poppy Jasper's red spots within the colorful Jasper matrix give it the appearance of a field of poppies. It symbolizes remembrance. Its energizing effect can be gentle or intense. Jasper was sacred to the native peoples of America and has always been known as a stone of protection. Poppy Jasper is particularly useful for repelling stalkers and releasing the ties of previous relationships.

HEALING POWER

Poppy Jasper is believed to regulate excessive bleeding, whether from wounds or menstrual flow. It is an excellent energizer in situations that call for a stronger flow of Qi through the body or when the pulse needs to be stabilized. Placed over the liver or bile duct, Poppy Jasper dissolves energetic blockages. Placed over the base and sacral chakras, it is said to counteract impotence, assist birth, and help release psychological causes that inhibit orgasm. Poppy Jasper placed over the fallopian tubes assists conception when psychosomatic blockages in the tubes inhibit the sperm's movement or when the sperm themselves are energetically sluggish. Poppy Jasper calms excessive libido and also clears frustration from unrequited lust. Conversely, it stimulates passion and strengthens a depleted libido.

   Your pet can wear Poppy Jasper as an amulet against dis-ease (enclose the stone in a strong wire wrap so your pet doesn't swallow it). You can distantly heal an animal by placing the stone over the appropriate organs and chakras on the owner's body. In many animals, dis-ease is psychosomatic; the animal takes on the owner's toxic feelings, blockages, and projections. If a disease is psychosomatic, healing the owner heals the animal. Subtle dis-ease, which ultimately becomes physical, may result if the animal absorbs energies that would be detrimental to its owner; for example, cats may choose to sit in a place of strong geopathic or electromagnetic stress and absorb the resulting disharmony, protecting their owners. Gridding around an animal's sleeping place with large Poppy Jasper may be beneficial—the stones need frequent cleansing and may have to be supported with Smoky Quartz or Black Tourmaline.

TRANSFORMATIONAL POWER

Use Poppy Jasper if you are faced with an unjust situation or need to deal with a problem before it becomes too advanced. By insisting that you be honest with yourself about the source of the situation, it helps to strengthen your assertive qualities and gives you the stamina to persevere until a satisfactory solution is found.

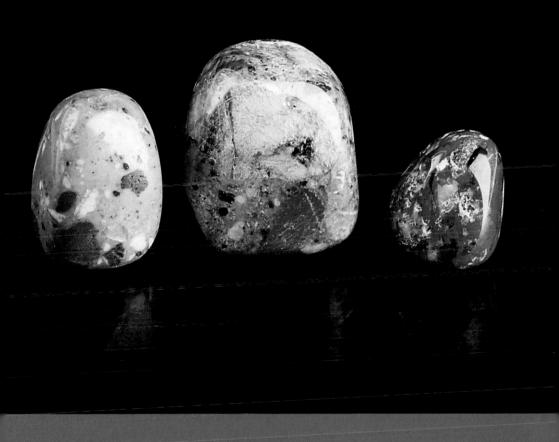

Kept in your pocket or under
your pillow, Poppy Jasper
spceds recovery during illness,
convalescence, or hospitalization.

Preseli Bluestone

- **Chakra correspondences:** Soma, earth, base, sacral, past life, higher heart (thymus)
- **Physiological correspondences:** Hippocampus, neurotransmitters, throat, ears, and immune and electrical systems
- **Vibration:** Earthy and high

LEGENDARY POWER

Carrying immense healing energy, Preseli Bluestone radiates power and forms a doorway to other dimensions. The central ring at Stonehenge is formed from Preseli Bluestone, a spotted dolerite transported more than two hundred miles from Pembrokeshire in Wales—an incredible feat as the wheel had not yet been invented. Legend tells us the stones were flown from Ireland by Merlin, King Arthur's magician, but the stones are five thousand years older, and originally formed Stonehenge's outer circle. This outer circle, now known as the Aubrey holes, mapped the phases and eclipses of the long moon cycle—and Bluestone is a stone of dreaming and far memory. Tradition says sick individuals were passed between the stones for healing purposes. A new, even earlier Bluestone circle has recently been discovered nearby, which archaeologists believe linked the domain of the dead (the area around Stonehenge) with that of the living (Durrington Walls). Bluestone, therefore, has an ancient connection to the ancestors and is excellent for multidimensional journeying. It links to the magical, archetypal Merlin energy that brings out the shaman in everyone.

Connected to currents in the Earth, Bluestone has a strong magnetic charge that can be harnessed for Earth healing and to access ancient knowledge. Bluestone increases sensitivity to vibrations, heightening awareness of crystal, meridian, or sound frequencies. Some Bluestone is lithographic (see Granite, page 96).

HEALING POWER

Balancing the meridians and restoring energetic harmony, Bluestone creates unshakable core stability for the physical and energetic bodies. Placed over the thymus gland, it energetically strengthens the subtle immune system. At the base of the skull, it harmonizes the brain stem and activates the hippocampus, an inner compass that orients you in the physical world. A powerful Earth harmonizer, Bluestone ameliorates the effects of electromagnetic smog and light pollution. It facilitates deep karmic healing under the guidance of an experienced practitioner. Combining Bluestone with chalk (on the left in this photo) produces a powerful battery to combat energy depletion in the physical body or the Earth.

TRANSFORMATIONAL POWER

If you have lost your sense of spiritual direction, Bluestone reconnects you to your life purpose. It focuses your mind and strengthens willpower, helping you face challenges with equanimity. If part of your soul or emotional energy remains entangled in the past, Bluestone frees you to live in the present moment. (Note: If a headache develops when using Bluestone, turn it or yourself so the stone's magnetic resonance aligns with the Earth's.)

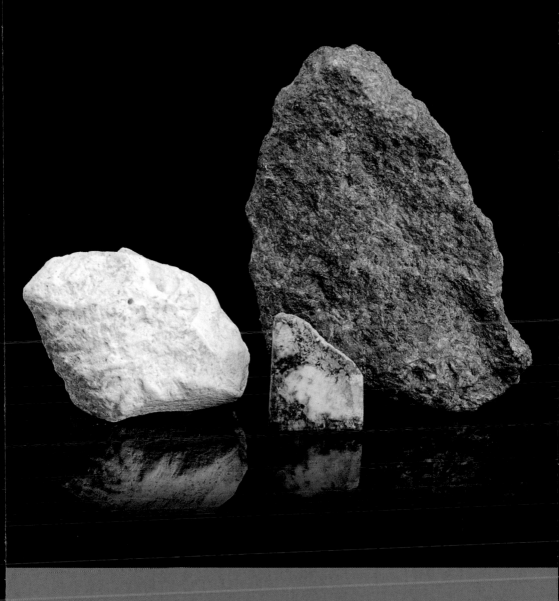

Place Bluestone on your soma chakra or base of the skull to transcend time, access past or future, and reconnect to your ancient knowing.

Quantum Quattro

- **Chakra correspondences:** All chakras, particularly higher heart (thymus), heart seed, third eye, solar plexus
- **Physiological correspondences:** Cellular and intercellular structures, blood and circulation, pancreas and insulin production, thyroid and metabolic processes, immune system, ears, lungs, heart, digestive tract, DNA
- **Vibration:** High

LEGENDARY POWER

Although the Quantum Quattro combination has only recently come into crystal lore, its component parts are among the earliest known healing stones. Malachite has long been reputed to protect against evil spirits and is an efficient cleansing stone, as is Smoky Quartz. Chrysocolla enhances personal power and conducts energy, as do Dioptase and Shattuckite, which also amplify the aura. All these stones repair subtle DNA information, switching off genetically transmitted energetic codes for dis-ease. Quantum Quattro provides enormous protection for the soul. As with all synergistic stones, the power of the whole is much greater than the sum of its parts. It emits a palpable energy field that harmonizes the human energy field to the quantum. This stone enhances your manifestation powers—whatever you visualize, you bring into being.

Quantum Quattro reminds us that healing must not involve judgment, either of ourselves or others. Judgment, or feelings of superiority, contaminates the healing process, lowering the vibrations of all concerned rather than creating equilibrium at a higher frequency.

HEALING POWER

Quantum Quattro works with the quantum field to rebalance and recalibrate, creating healing on multiple levels and dimensions. A master healer, the stone may aid virtually all conditions. Crystal workers use it to regularize metabolic functioning and repair subtle genetic programming, optimizing twelve-strand DNA activation and clearing patterns of dis-ease from the ancestral line. It may also combat fungal infections.

Quantum Quattro gently completes a healing crisis or catharsis provoked by more intense stones as it facilitates transmutation of the underlying energies. Carry this crystal as a prophylactic against pain and disease. At an emotional level, Quantum Quattro heals unresolved grief and the psychosomatic causes of dis-ease. It releases blocks to seeing clearly, hypnotic commands implanted in the present or other lifetimes, and karmic wounds or inner child issues. By drawing in unconditional love, it heals the pain of abandonment. This stone is an effective environmental healer, too.

TRANSFORMATIONAL POWER

Placing a Quantum Quattro on the solar plexus and third eye ensures that mind, body, and spirit work in harmony to facilitate the expansion process. During metaphysical work, Quantum Quattro heightens spiritual awareness. It supports kything and prevents the communicating spirit from taking permanent control. The crystal helps you work with focused intention for the highest good and lets you clearly see your path to quantum healing.

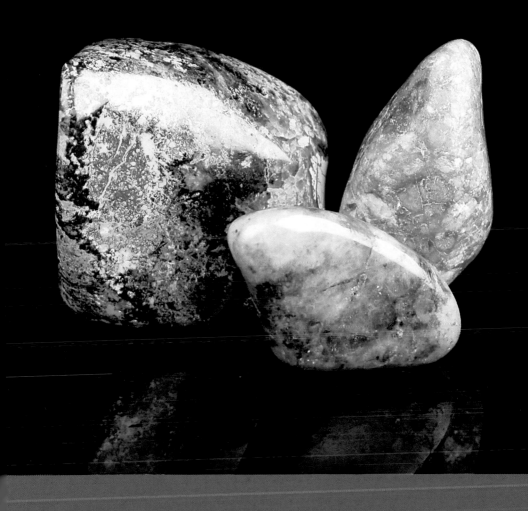

Grid Quantum Quattro around
a sick bed to bring the body
back into balance and encourage
the production of T cells by the
immune system.

Quartz

- **Chakra correspondences:** All chakras; purifies and expands the auric field
- **Physiological correspondences:** All systems and organs of the physical and subtle bodies, mineral assimilation
- **Vibration:** Earthy to exceptionally high, depending on type; may be both

LEGENDARY POWER

The indigenous people of America placed Quartz in the cradles of newborns to connect them with the Earth. Large Quartz points were found in an eight thousand-year-old Egyptian temple. The eighth-century B.C.E. Greek priest Onomacritus tells us that anyone entering a temple with the crystal in hand was certain to have his prayers answered, as the gods cannot resist its power. Quartz was used throughout the ancient world for scrying and to heighten metaphysical abilities. The Maya dowsed for water with it. Apollonius of Tyrea, a first-century Christian mystic, had a crystal ball that apparently allowed him to appear and disappear at will—he allegedly did so in the presence of Caesar.

Pliny bemoans the fact that many pieces of Quartz are impaired by defects, such as "rough solder-like excrescences," occlusions of water, cloudy or "salt-spots," bright red rust, and internal fibers—all prized by crystal workers today for the properties they add to the underlying crystal.

Quartz is silica, the most abundant element in the Earth and the human body. An example of "as above, so below," silica is essential for healthy, well-oxygenated cells; it is one of the building blocks of the immune system and our planet. A master healer, Quartz amplifies energy and optimizes health. The medieval Ashmole lapidary states that Quartz quenched thirst and made a man "lecherous and kend."

HEALING POWER

The ancients dipped Quartz in water to charge the water with magical healing power. In Pliny's day, doctors cauterized wounds with a crystal ball through which the sun's rays were focused to generate heat. Held away from the body, Quartz healed blisters.

Quartz brings the body into balance and energetically ameliorates any condition. Among its benefits are said to be regulation of blood pressure, reoxygenation of tissue, and regeneration of cells. It energetically strengthens metabolism, blood vessels, and elasticity of joints and connective tissue. Anti-inflammatory, it removes heat. This crystal breaks through blockages, removes toxins, and reattunes the body's inner vibrational structure.

TRANSFORMATIONAL POWER

Quartz holds a dynamic hologram of the soul and universal knowledge. The indigenous people of America refer to Quartz as the brain cells of Mother Earth, and this abundant crystal seems to instinctively know what is required. By attuning to your frequency, it transmutes negativity, amplifies energy, adjusts your vibrational field, and raises your consciousness. This deep soul cleanser removes the seeds of karmic dis-ease, detoxifies the emotional field, and balances your mind.

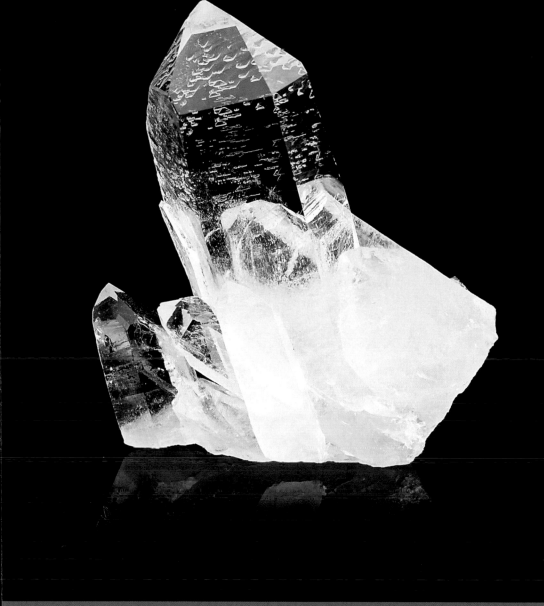

Place Quartz wherever
healing is needed. It restores
your whole being to energetic
harmony and wholeness.

Que Sera (Llanite/Llanoite)

- **Chakra correspondences:** Earth star, base, sacral, stellar gateway; activates the higher sacral chakra in the dantien
- **Physiological correspondences:** Subtle energy systems and meridians of the subtle and physical bodies, all the organs and systems of the physical body
- **Vibration:** Earthy and simultaneously extremely high

LEGENDARY POWER

A synergistic conglomerate from Brazil, Que Sera contains blue quartz, feldspar, calcite, kaolinite, iron, magnetite, leucozone, and clinozoisite. It holds the combined power of these constituents. The stone links to the power of the megaforces that brought our multidimensional universe into being, and which still drive cosmic evolution. Like a battery, Que Sera activates your own power. With this stone, you truly create your own reality. Llanite Rhyolite (Llanoite Granite) from Texas is energetically similar, although at an earthier vibration, with the same blue and pink inclusions. (See Aswan Granite, page 96.)

HEALING POWER

A powerful carrier of Qi, Que Sera recharges and balances the meridians and organs of the subtle and physical bodies. Place it wherever dis-ease or depletion exists. The stone activates neurotransmitters to optimize the energetic circuit—you feel as though your body has been plugged into an electric power source. Que Sera helps a healer see into the recipient's energy matrix, highlighting areas of dis-ease. Place the stone over a site for a few moments to dissolve dis-ease and restore the body's cellular and energetic structure. It can also serve as a dowsing rod—it twitches as it moves over places that need healing. Grid this stone to shield against electromagnetic smog, including Wi-Fi emanations that can create dis-ease in sensitive people.

TRANSFORMATIONAL POWER

Que Sera lets you stand in your own power. It releases you from self-imposed obliga-tions, especially those you unconsciously assumed so the world would perceive you as "a good person." The stone teaches that service given in this way is actually selfish and self-serving, and does not enhance the greater good. If you take the burdens of the world on your shoulders and find it impossible to say no when asked to do even more, keep Que Sera in your pocket. The transformation will free you to be of real service to those around you. If you dwell on problems, this crystal helps you find constructive solutions.

Que Sera means "what will be," but with this stone the future definitely is yours to cocreate. It attunes you to the Akashic Record of your soul's purpose and shows all pos-sible pathways. Pointing out the long way and the direct route, it encourages you to take the one most appropriate for your evolution. With Que Sera, there are no mistakes, only learning experiences. How fast you learn is up to you—it can be instantaneous.

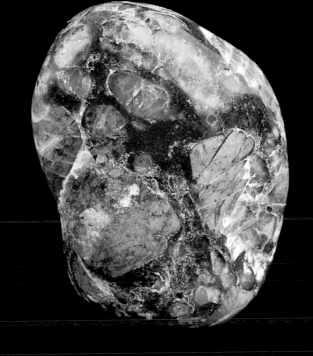

Place Que Sera at the higher sacral chakra within the dantien and breathe deeply to turn on a truly awesome personal powerhouse.

Rhodochrosite

- **Chakra correspondences:** Heart, higher heart (thymus), heart seed, soma; clears solar plexus and base chakras
- **Physiological correspondences:** Eyes; kidneys; lungs; thyroid gland; circulatory, metabolic, and urogenital systems
- **Vibration:** Earthy to high, depending on whether it is opaque or gem

LEGENDARY POWER

The stone of the compassionate heart, Rhodochrosite symbolizes selfless love. It lets you recognize the divine within yourself. It was created when white manganese dissolved with carbonate dripped into cavities, giving the stone its swirls of pink, red, and white. Rhodochrosite was sacred to the Incas, who called it Inca Rose and believed it was the solidified blood of their ancestral kings and queens. In a cave deep under the Andes, the heart of Mother Earth beats once every two hundred years. It is a Rhodochrosite heart-shaped boulder that has been sacred to the local people for millennia.

The Alfonso lapidary describes an astringent stone with cleansing and drying properties called *Almartac*, believed to be Rhodochrosite. It calmed itching and, mixed with wax, healed ulcers, cleared away putrid flesh, and reduced pain. We are given a tantalizing hint that it was used in alchemy, but the secret is not included in that book.

The Sweet Home mine in Alma, Colorado, produces rare and exceedingly beautiful red Rhodochrosite, found nowhere else on Earth.

HEALING POWER

Rhodochrosite contains manganese, an important physiological constituent of the body with a powerful antioxidant and metabolic function. Required for correct bone development, manganese is also necessary for repairing tissue and assimilation of minerals. However, manganese can be toxic in large quantities. This may be why Rhodochrosite has such profound healing properties, as it is impossible to give too strong an energetic dose when using the crystal as it brings about balance.

Traditionally, Rhodochrosite assists the heart and circulatory systems, and removes irritants from the lungs. Placed at the base of the skull, it may dilate blood vessels, relieve tension migraines, and stabilize blood pressure. Gem Rhodochrosite has been used to heal psychosomatic causes of cancers and other dis-eases, and to reprogram the etheric blueprint to a healthier pattern.

TRANSFORMATIONAL POWER

Rhodochrosite opens the compassionate heart and fills it with unconditional love. Gem Rhodochrosite has a higher vibration, opening the heart seed chakra for an infusion of divine love. This crystal is excellent for past-life healing and, placed over the heart, for gently disentangling the ties of outgrown relationships. On the soma chakra, it facilitates reading the Akashic Record to ascertain the purpose of your present incarnation.

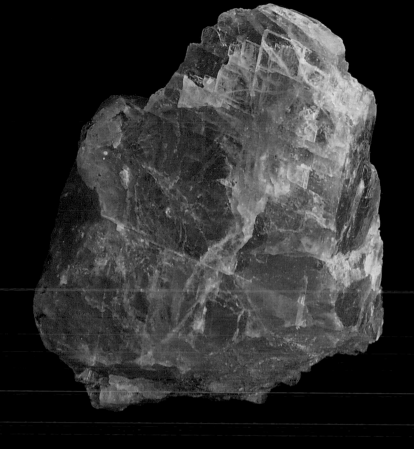

Program Rhodochrosite to attract
a twin flame, someone with whom
you can share unconditional love
and mutual support.

Rhodonite

- **Chakra correspondences:** Heart, higher heart (thymus), heart seed, solar plexus
- **Physiological correspondences:** Heart, skin, nervous and respiratory systems
- **Vibration:** Earthy

LEGENDARY POWER

Named after the Greek word for rosy, Rhodonite's often intense bicolor comes from black and white manganese. It was formed into platters and given as a royal wedding gift by the czars of Russia, which fits its reputation as a stone that nurtures love.

Rhodonite is prized for its ability to instill emotional balance and heal emotional wounds, particularly those lodged in the heart chakra, gently releasing abuse and self-destructive tendencies. It fosters brotherhood and lets you see both sides of an issue to reach conciliation. This crystal turns back insults and makes you aware that revenge and retaliation are wastes of energy; it is particularly useful in dangerous situations. Holding it calms you during trauma and ameliorates panic attacks. Rhodonite supports you during any challenging situation, helping you stay heart-centered no matter what occurs.

HEALING POWER

Rhodonite contains manganese, which acts as an effective wound healer, relieves the itching of insect bites, and encourages bone growth. Traditionally used to calm ulcers, Rhodonite may aid autoimmune dis-eases such as arthritis. It is said to be anti-inflammatory for joints and calms the lungs, easing emphysema. Placed behind the ears, it fine-tunes auditory vibrations to assist hearing and relieve tinnitus. Crystal workers use the stone or Rhodonite-infused water as a first aid remedy for trauma or shock at physical, emotional, mental, and/or spiritual levels.

Place Rose Quartz on the heart chakra, Tugtupite on the heart seed, Rhodochrosite over the higher heart, and Rhodonite on the solar plexus to heal heartbreak and open the higher heart and heart seed chakras to unconditional love. Lying in a Rhodonite grid also dissolves memories of abuse, emotional scars, and feelings that may have festered for many lifetimes, replacing them with love and forgiveness for yourself and others.

TRANSFORMATIONAL POWER

Rhodonite teaches that emotions are responses you make to feelings that are neutral until your mind forms an attitude about them. Such judgments can create an emotional stranglehold, especially when passed on from lifetime to lifetime. Rhodonite assists emotional recalibration, so you no longer react the way you did before. You can then offer yourself and others unconditional love and acceptance. If you lack trust in yourself, Rhodonite encourages self-confidence and assists you in fulfilling your highest potential. By transmuting lust and excessive libido into a loving exchange of passionate sexual energy, Rhodonite helps lovers achieve tantric union.

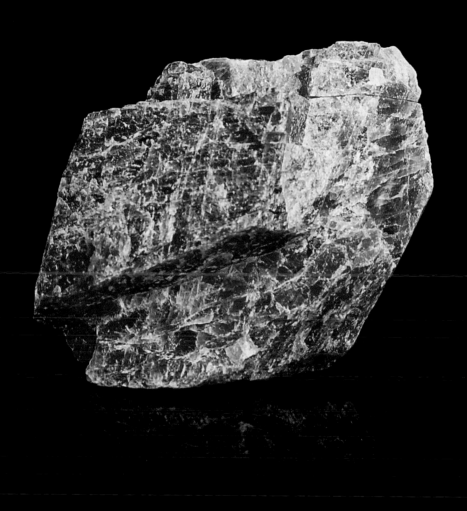

Place Rhodonite on your
heart to allow feelings to simply
pass through you, acknowledging
them, letting them flow, until
they move on.

Rose Quartz

- **Chakra correspondences:** Heart, higher heart (thymus), heart seed
- **Physiological correspondences:** Heart, blood, circulation, thymus gland, lungs, adrenals, skin, brain stem, and reproductive and lymphatic systems
- **Vibration:** Earthy and high

LEGENDARY POWER

Rose Quartz has long been known as the stone of unconditional love. In the Middle Ages, it decorated the St. Wenceslaus Chapel in Prague. This may have had specific symbolism as Wenceslaus was the much-loved patron saint of the Czech Republic.

Rose Quartz heals emotions and transforms relationships with yourself and others, drawing in love and harmony. Hold this crystal of auric and heart protection to bring loving vibes into your heart and subtle etheric bodies. At a metaphysical level, Rose Quartz stimulates the third eye, strengthening scrying power and opening clairvoyance to the finest levels of guidance.

HEALING POWER

Prized by crystal workers for its effect on the heart, Rose Quartz releases unexpressed emotions and underlying heartache that create psychosomatic dis-ease and which may affect fertility. Under the principle of sympathetic magic, its deep pink color strengthens the blood and circulation system, improving energy flow and removing impurities. This gentle crystal energetically harmonizes the brain, realigning neurotransmitters and opening new neural pathways and may assist dementia, Alzheimer's, and Parkinson's. Placed over the higher heart (thymus) chakra, it may calm asthma attacks and other breathing difficulties.

TRANSFORMATIONAL POWER

During midlife crisis or traumatic times, Rose Quartz stabilizes emotions. It lets you look objectively at situations and keeps you from becoming emotionally overwhelmed. By dissolving guilt and bitterness, this crystal teaches you to love and accept yourself, forgive the past, and live from your heart. If you are unable to recognize where emotion is locked into your body, hold Rose Quartz, inhale deeply, and then exhale. Stay in the stillness of the out-breath and let your body tell you where it feels the tension. Breathe again to draw in healing love and direct it to the site with the power of your mind or by placing the crystal over the spot.

The rarer Elestial Rose Quartz and Gemmy Rose Quartz draw unconditional love down to Earth. They remind you that you can always empower yourself through positive choices and expressing unconditional love from a compassionate heart. Laid on the higher heart and heart seed chakras, these stones transport you into the heart of the universe—where there is no karma, no past, and no future, just the immediate present—and from there into the temple of your own heart where everything is love.

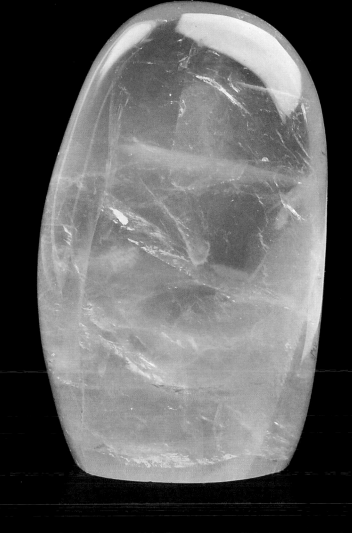

If you feel disempowered
or unloved, hold Rose Quartz
and remind yourself of a time
when you felt positive and potent,
loved and accepted.

Ruby in Zoisite (Anyolite)

- **Chakra correspondences:** Base, sacral, heart, crown
- **Physiological correspondences:** Testicles, ovaries, heart, circulatory system, pancreas, lungs, sleeping disorders, stress, acidification balance
- **Vibration:** Earthy and high

LEGENDARY POWER

Combination stones interweave the vibrations of both, and Ruby in Zoisite exemplifies crystal cooperation. Ruby symbolizes all things hot, active, and passionate—vigor, lust, libido, aggression, assertion, machismo—but Zoisite is a temperate, selfless stone.

Our ancestors carried Ruby amulets to ward off war, danger, and aggression. Greek legend tells us a woman who treated a lame stork kindly was rewarded with a Ruby that lit up her room at night. Astarte, the Mesopotamian goddess of fertility, motherhood, and war, owned a Ruby that illuminated her temple with supernatural light. Astarte watched over the souls of the dead, visible as stars in the heavens. So, Ruby has long been associated with kindness and nurturing, death, and bringing light into dark places.

Put these qualities into a matrix of Zoisite, and you have a combination for profound emotional and spiritual transformation. Ruby in Zoisite transmutes grief, giving comfort to the bereaved. Zoisite also helps you speak your truth, blocking the influence of others; Ruby contributes courage to speak out against injustice.

HEALING POWER

Chinese medicine sees grief as affecting the lungs. Ruby in Zoisite is useful when stress or grief creates dis-ease or congestion. It encourages you to talk about emotions and losses underlying depression and lethargy. The ancients used Ruby to treat fever, inflammation, and hemorrhage because both crystal and patient were hot and red. In 1584, Ivan the Terrible stated that Ruby improved memory and "clarified congealed blood, corrupt blood." Crystal workers use Ruby to detoxify blood and blood-rich organs, and to invigorate the excretory organs, heart, and circulatory system. Ruby in Zoisite's powerful amplification effect on the energetic body strengthens the aura, bringing about multidimensional cellular healing. It also promotes the will to recover.

TRANSFORMATIONAL POWER

Ruby symbolizes the fires that temper the soul's resilience. A catalyst for core soul healing, Ruby in Zoisite activates soul memories and brings emotional blockages to the surface for transmutation. Turning self-destructive emotions, such as anger or rage, into an assertive will advances your life with compassion and care for others. Ruby in Zoisite helps you see the purpose behind losses you experience in your life. It opens your compassion for others undergoing similar pain. The stone helps you think positively and live with passion. When holding Ruby in Zoisite, you experience interconnectedness with All That Is while appreciating your own individuality. (See Tanzanite/Lavender-Blue Zoisite, page 202).

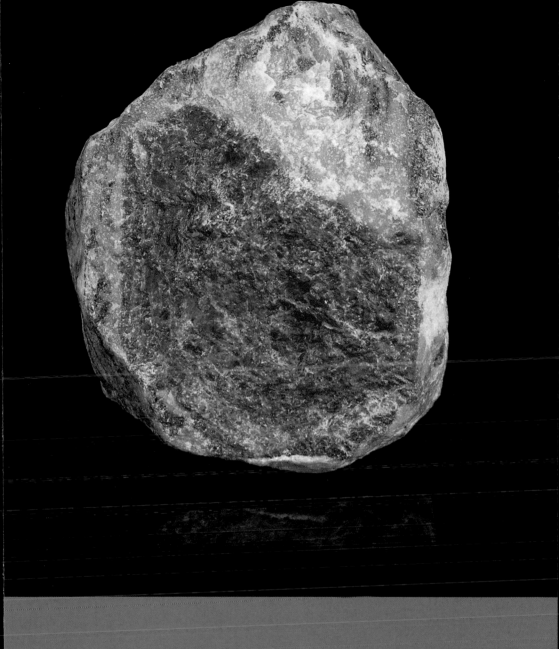

Wear Ruby in Zoisite over your heart if you are grieving. It brings spiritual comfort and release and attracts new passion into your life.

Rutilated Quartz

- **Chakra correspondences:** Harmonizes and aligns all chakras, including the soul star and stellar gateway, with the aura
- **Physiological correspondences:** Thyroid and thymus glands, cellular structure, blood vessels, and urogenital and respiratory systems
- **Vibration:** Earthy and high

LEGENDARY POWER

Rutilated Quartz's power comes from Rutile, the purifying and protective mineral included at its core, synergized with Quartz. This Quartz is often known as Angel's Hair because of the fine strands of titanium dioxide (Rutile) that form within the crystal and amplify the basic Quartz energy. In crystal lore, this stone connects to the highest angelic frequencies. It is named after the Latin *rutilus*, which means "red," but Rutile is also found in an ethereal golden form. Angel's Hair could be likened to modern string theory, which describes the universe in terms of complex multidimensional strings, rather than the restricted, three-dimensional particle theory. Supersymmetrical strings create metaphysical links, such as portals, membranes, and higher-dimensional objects, with forces similar to electromagnetism. These refer directly to the properties of Rutilated Quartz, which has the perfect balance of cosmic light and creative power.

HEALING POWER

Rutilated Quartz draws off negative energy during a chakra sweep and provides a firm foundation for new energetic patterns to be imprinted into the cells. In past-life healing, it promotes insight into the core issue. It also reveals if a particular dis-ease has been taken on deliberately as a soul-learning experience and provides support to continue with it.

Crystal workers use Rutilated Quartz to energetically re-balance the thyroid, heal the lungs, and stimulate cellular growth. Placed on the jaw, muscles, or abdomen it energetically absorbs toxicity from mercury-amalgam fillings. At an emotional level, Rutilated Quartz heals the past and dissolves the deeper causes of depression and psychiatric disorders, such as phobias or anxiety. An efficient Earth healer for geopathic stress, it soaks up electromagnetic smog.

TRANSFORMATIONAL POWER

Rutilated Quartz purifies toxic thoughts and constrictive emotions, releasing the past so barriers to spiritual evolution are dissolved and soul purpose comes into play. Placed over the third eye, it opens your metaphysical sight and enhances your intuition. Using Rutilated Quartz on the chakras connects "power rods" that coexist between subtle chakra points and the lightbody; this activation vastly accelerates spiritual growth. Placed on the third eye, Rutilated Quartz amplifies the power of thought so your thoughts are projected out into the world in tangible, solidified form—it can bring you all you desire. Use this crystal with care and consideration for others, for if the power is misused selfishly or abusively, it will backfire.

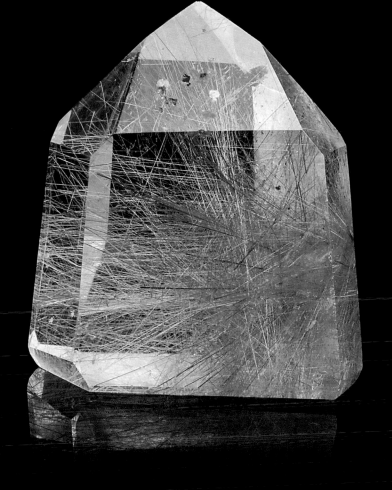

Place energetically vibrant
Rutilated Quartz on your solar plexus
or over the thymus to heighten the life
force and heal chronic dis-eases and
sexual dysfunction.

Sapphire

- **Chakra correspondences:** Third eye
- **Physiological correspondences:** Eyes, endocrine glands, circulatory system, cells
- **Vibration:** High

LEGENDARY POWER

Sapphire means "Beloved of Saturn" in Sanskrit and the stone is one of the great metaphysical healing gems of Vedic astrology. According to Hindu legend, Saturn was the first planet to appear out of the void, and Star Sapphire, with its strikingly bright star formation, symbolizes the emergence of light out of darkness.

In the sixteenth century, Ivan the Terrible delighted in Sapphire because "it preserveth, and inceaseth courage, joys, the heart, is pleasing to all the vital senses, precious and very sovereign for the eyes, cheers the sight, takes away bloodshot, strengthens the muscles and the strings thereof."

Traditionally, the gem was presented to Bishops of the Roman Catholic Church to symbolize their vow of chastity and to retain their innocence and purity. In the language of gemstones, Sapphire still signifies innocence, constancy, truth, and virtue. It is considered to be a crystal of endurance and wisdom. In ancient Mesopotamia, people believed the heavens consisted of crystalline spheres—an idea that continued into Renaissance times. In Ezekiel, Sapphire forms the throne of God; in Revelations, it is one of the foundation stones of the New Jerusalem, echoing the belief that it was one of the stones in the Breastplate of the Jewish High Priest. A stone of Archangels Metatron, angel of integration, and Zadkiel, the comforter, Sapphire rules over the Seraphic realm.

HEALING POWER

In the lapidaries of the Middle Ages, Sapphire was reputed to heal the eyes, and way back into history, it was also used for diseases of the blood. Crystal healers today still use Sapphire to improve the elasticity of veins, heal blood disorders, and regulate overactive glands and systems of the body. Sapphire-infused water can be used to bathe the eyes to ensure crystal-clear sight.

TRANSFORMATIONAL POWER

Sapphires come in many colors, and each has its own unique properties. Blue Sapphire encourages you to seek out spiritual truth. Pink Sapphire draws into your life exactly what you need to evolve. Yellow Sapphire is a crystal of abundance that attracts wealth and stimulates insight. Black Sapphire centers and protects. Star Sapphire provides you with a guiding star during the course of your life, supported by the three cross bars of faith, hope, and destiny.

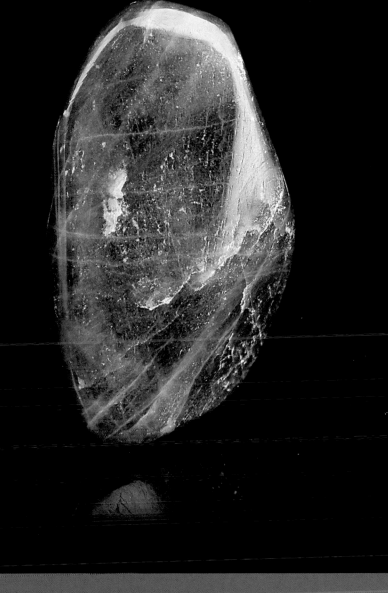

Wearing Sapphire reminds you
that the soul is pure and innocent
with perfect intention and moral
integrity. It brings you peace of
mind and serenity.

Satyaloka™ and Satyamani™ Quartz

- **Chakra correspondences:** Crown, soul star, stellar gateway, and beyond; cleanses and reattunes the aura

- **Physiological correspondences:** These Quartzes work beyond the physical body; they amplify the vibrations of other healing stones

- **Vibration:** Exceptionally high

LEGENDARY POWER

Buddhists say Quartz is one of the seven precious substances, and Satyaloka Quartz's vibration has been raised by people from the Satyaloka Monastery in South India (now closed). It is said that the greatest number of enlightened souls on the planet live nearby, specifically to assist in world consciousness-raising and to bring enlightenment to those ready to receive it. Spiritual light is infused into the basic Quartz before it is sent out into the world. Satyamani has been similarly attuned. These spiritual power-houses create profound union with the divine and open the highest levels of mystical consciousness. We can gain an idea of how this transformation of the crystal is achieved from a passage in the *Kalpa Sutra*, an ancient sacred book of the Jains:

> *Then he [the god] transformed himself through his magical power of transformation, and stretched himself out for numerous Yoganas like a staff, during which he seized jewels. Of this precious material he rejected the gross particles and retained the subtle particles . . . he [then] passed with that excellent, hasty, trembling, active, impetuous, victorious, exalted and quick divine motion of the gods right through numberless continents and oceans.*

For hundreds of years, people living around Satyaloka have reported intense spiritual and mystical experiences, out-of-body journeying, and heightened psychic sensitivity. This metaphysical energy has been infused into the stones. Satyaloka means "the abode of truth" or "the descent of light to Earth." Satyaloka is now categorized as Azeztulite (see page 46).

HEALING POWER

These Quartzes work beyond the physical body to raise the frequencies of the subtle bodies and effect multidimensional, holistic soul healing. Satyaloka and Satyamani infuse light when placed on either side of the head, level with the past life chakras with Nirvana Quartz (page 136) on the soul star chakra a foot above the head. A Smoky Elestial or other grounding stone at the feet anchors the new vibrations into the physical plane.

In a planetary healing grid, these stones—especially in combination with other high-vibration stones such as Ajoite, Azeztulite, and Trigonic—open the Earth's higher crown chakras and infuse divine light into the Earth's matrix.

TRANSFORMATIONAL POWER

Satyamani and Satyaloka Quartz effect enlightenment—quite literally. They bring light into the physical plane and open the illumined mind to an influx of pure spirit. These holy stones create an interface between the soul and the physical body, ensuring that you never walk your spiritual path alone.

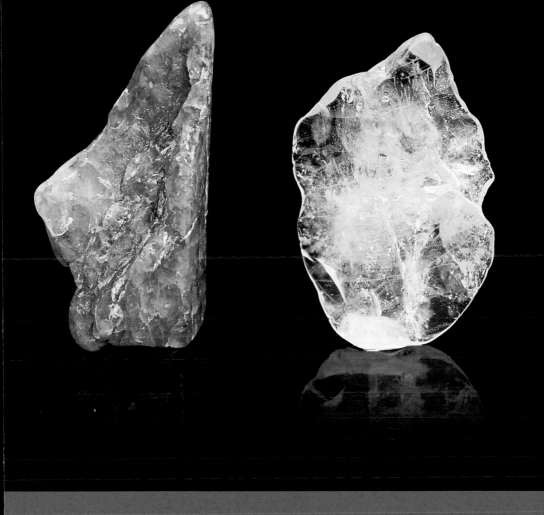

Placed on either side of your head, these Quartzes create an inner temple of light and facilitate direct communication with the divine.

Selenite

- **Chakra correspondences:** Crown, soul star, stellar gateway, and beyond
- **Physiological correspondences:** Spinal column, joints, breasts, nerves, puberty, menopause; the most profound healing occurs at an energetic rather than physical level
- **Vibration:** High to exceptionally high

LEGENDARY POWER

Selenite stands at the threshold between spirit and matter. A Kabbalistic creation myth tells us that before the universe existed, God was everywhere, but he had to inhale to create space for our world. Realizing he was not present in creation, he fashioned vessels of divine light to populate the universe, but they shattered. Carrying that light, Selenite's task is to reunite the shards of the divine with their source.

Selenite was traditionally used for scrying. An eleventh-century lapidary says Selenite grows with the waxing moon and diminishes with the waning one. The Alfonso lapidary says if the stone is hung on a tree, the fruit will grow and ripen rapidly.

HEALING POWER

In ancient Mesopotamia, Selenite kept sickrooms free from evil spirits. The "Ritual for Curing a Sick Man" reveals, "The selenite and the bitumen which they [the priests] smear on the door of the sick man, the selenite is Ninurta. The bitumen is Asakku. Ninurta pursues Asakku." Ninurta is Saturn, a good guy, and Asakku an evil deity. The spell says Asakku was caught in a ritually created net, much as modern crystal workers use a Selenite grid to constrain a destructive entity.

The Alfonso lapidary tells us Selenite cured epilepsy; wearing it prevented attacks. Today crystal workers use Selenite to ameliorate detrimental effects of dental amalgam and free radicals. Green Selenite may delay aging of the skeleton and skin. Fishtail Selenite supports nerves and neural pathways. Peach Selenite assists puberty and menopause. Placing Blue Selenite on the third eye chakra silences mental chatter and opens the third eye. Pure white Selenite is an excellent auric cleanser and healer. All Selenite acts as an emotional stabilizer that calms mood swings.

TRANSFORMATIONAL POWER

Selenite accesses angelic consciousness and brings divine light into everything it touches. White or Golden Selenite forms a bridge for the lightbody, facilitating expansion of consciousness and integration of the divine. A powerful transmutor for emotional energy, Selenite releases core feelings behind psychosomatic illnesses and emotional blockages. Connected to Persephone, Greek Queen of the Underworld, Peach Selenite shines light into dark places to help you understand your inner processes and integrate shadow qualities. It also facilitates female rites of passage, such as puberty and menopause, encouraging reconnection to the wise feminine divine power. (Note: Selenite dissolves in water. Cleanse in brown rice and re-empower in moonlight.)

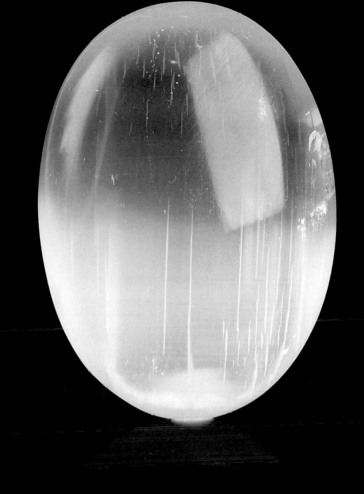

Hold Selenite above your head.
Feel it radiating divine light
through your whole being,
illuminating your inner temple and
connecting you to All That Is.

Septarian

- **Chakra correspondences:** Earth star, base; synthesizes third eye, throat, and heart chakras
- **Physiological correspondences:** Metabolism, skin, heart, intestines, kidneys, blood, cellular memory, mineral absorption
- **Vibration:** Earthy

LEGENDARY POWER

Seventy million years ago, volcanic activity under the sea killed marine life. As it fell to the seabed and decayed, mud balls formed filled with concretions of Calcite (the yellow portion of Septarian), Aragonite (the brown lines), and Limestone (the gray coating). The balls cracked in a distinctive formation of seven fissures radiating out from the center. The resulting stones look rather like turtle shells. The nodules were called *Septarian* after *septum*, the Latin for seven or *saeptum*, a wall or enclosure. The combination is extremely powerful. Aragonite's (page 38) devic energy is an excellent Earth healer, and nurturing Calcite supports personal and planetary growth. Septarian encourages caring for the environment and everything on our planet.

If you speak in public, use Septarian to capture the audience's attention and let each person feel addressed individually. The process becomes effortless communication at the profoundest level. Septarian also makes you aware of the power of speech and its effect, not only on the listener but also within your own body. What the psyche perceives, the body conceives. Changing how you speak, the language with which you put your ideas across, can dramatically change your world. This grounding stone helps you speak only in the positive, present tense as it takes your attention away from negativities in the past. Septarian is also beneficial in sound healing.

HEALING POWER

Meditating with Septarian can illuminate the underlying causes of dis-ease. The crystal focuses the body's self-healing ability, detecting and dissolving energy blockages. It energetically rebalances the metabolism and reprograms cellular memory. Highly effective against seasonal affective disorder (SAD), it may reduce swelling and support structures and organs within the body. It also energetically assists drug users during detox and maintains strength of purpose thereafter.

Grid Septarian around a child's bed to prevent nightmares or to ameliorate night twitches in adults. Septarian stimulates physical growth in children; in adults it keeps joints flexible. It also calms the intestines and nervous system.

Septarian supports NLP sessions and is useful for tapping points in EFT and other meridian-based techniques. It repatterns the new behavior and beliefs into neurotransmitters and cellular memory.

TRANSFORMATIONAL POWER

Septarian concretizes your ideas. The perfect stone for increasing creativity, it supports any endeavor and grounds your intention into everyday reality.

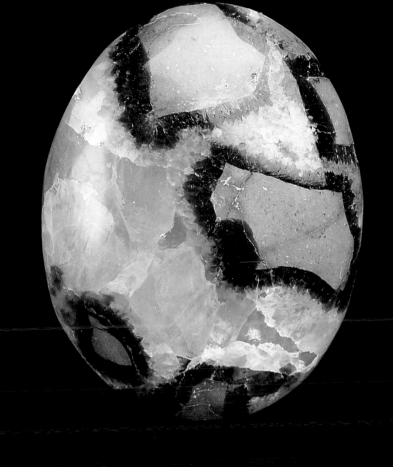

Keep a piece of Septarian with you when you speak in public—it helps you speak charismatically, with confidence and power.

Serpentine

- **Chakra correspondences:** Base, crown; purifies and energizes all chakras
- **Physiological correspondences:** Pancreas and insulin regulation, calcium and magnesium balance, detoxification and lymphatic processes, pain relief. Picrolite: adrenals, heart, endocrine system; Atlantisite: cellular memory, blood function
- **Vibration:** Earthy to high, depending on type

LEGENDARY POWER

With its distinctive likeness to snakeskin, Serpentine has a long tradition of protecting against snake and scorpion bites. Stones drew poison from wounds and the medieval *Peterborough Lapidary* comments on Serpentine's sweet smell, saying, "it is gode for venym." Used for medicine cups, it increased efficacy of a prescribed remedy. In ancient Egypt, Serpentine scarabs were interred with the dead to assist passage through the afterlife. Placed over the heart the inscription read: "I am reunited with the earth. I am not dead I am in Amenti. I am now a pure spirit for eternity."

Serpents have long symbolized divine power and wisdom. Place Serpentine on the base of the spine to raise kundalini "serpent power." Kundalini is a magical, tantric blending of masculine and feminine sexual currents, a subtle electromagnetic energy that potentizes chakras and ignites the flame of spiritual love, bringing about union with the divine. When awakened and passed upward through all the chakras, kundalini curls back to lie above the sacral chakra. In the dantien, it blends carnal desire, expanded consciousness, and a sense of personal power into a potent creative force.

Picrolite, dark green Serpentine, was used in prehistoric times as an Earth healer and protective amulet—it is still effective today, as is Atlantisite. This stone helps to access previous lives in Atlantis.

HEALING POWER

Serpentine was long prized for its healing virtue. Its reputed ability to control the flow of insulin in the body and to regulate the pancreas made it useful for healing diabetes, hypoglycemia, and hyperglycemia. It was also believed to eliminate parasites. Infinite Stone assists with between-lives karmic and soul healing, facilitating reintegration.

TRANSFORMATIONAL POWER

A powerful shamanic stone, Serpentine gives you a serpent's cunning when traveling in the underworld for soul retrieval and stimulates the magical skin shedding that facilitates shapeshifting and regeneration. It lends verbal cunning when you need to be particularly persuasive. Serpentine helps you understand the effects of past lives on the present, transforming negative qualities into positive gifts and recognizing the soul's hard-earned wisdom. Leopardskin Serpentine attunes you to the energy of Leopard and helps you reclaim lost power. If you misused your spiritual gifts in previous lives, Atlantisite re-empowers your soul. It assists in breaking patterns resulting from unwise choices or actions that lacked integrity.

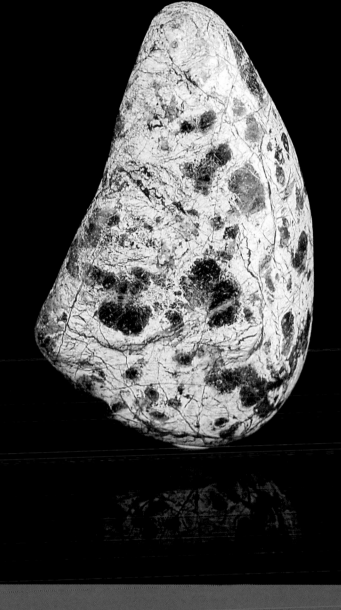

Place Serpentine over the
base chakra to stimulate kundalini
power, causing it to rise through
the central channel to the
higher chakras.

Shiva Lingam

- **Chakra correspondences:** Base and sacral; ignites all
- **Physiological correspondences:** Reproductive and electrical systems
- **Vibration:** Earthy and high

LEGENDARY POWER

Natural Shiva Lingam comes from the Narmada River in the Maridhata Mountains, one of the seven sacred sites of India. Its phallic shape and Quartz and Agate particles carry a powerful energetic charge and symbolize the union of opposites, a nonduality that extends beyond the physical world. Artificial Lingams are shaped from sandstone because legend says the goddess Parvati fashioned the first Lingam from sand to worship Lord Shiva. Sand represents the primal element of Earth, the phallus the primeval power of the male god, the soft texture the wise feminine goddess energy. The stone embodies the wisdom of the deities brought to Earth.

A Lingam also symbolizes the cosmic egg from which creation arose. According to another Indian legend, Shiva battled a fellow god over who had the greatest power. When Shiva won, a Lingam appeared in the sky. Therefore, Lingam symbolizes ultimate power. Both destroyer and renewer, Shiva represents the cycle of life, death, and rebirth. A Lingam teaches "this too will pass," and aids you in moving on. Additionally, Shiva is the god of mercy and compassion. Add a Lingam to a household altar for protection and to attract love into your home.

Sometimes Shiva is portrayed as "the Lord who is half woman," indicating that the power of the universe has masculine and feminine energy in equal measure. The bicolored Lingam represents male and female union and the alchemical marriage that merges inner masculine and feminine energies into androgynous power. This balance brings the body to a refined level of physical functioning, greater energetic resonance creating a stronger flow of Qi. A Lingam facilitates the kundalini rise that brings body and soul into unified enlightenment.

Use a Lingam to cut subtle ties with former partners, especially links through the chakras. It removes energetic hooks from the vagina. Because it enhances trust, it facilitates deeper union with your present partner through tantric magic, and can draw a relationship that brings sexual healing.

HEALING POWER

Lingam's healing power works with the reproductive organs to energetically stimulate potency and fertility. The stone overcomes memories of abuse and the underlying psychosomatic causes of inorgasmia. Placed over the uterus, it may relieve menstrual cramps.

TRANSFORMATIONAL POWER

Shiva Lingam releases you from the past and psychological patterns you have outgrown, particularly around sexual matters. It opens your creativity at every level.

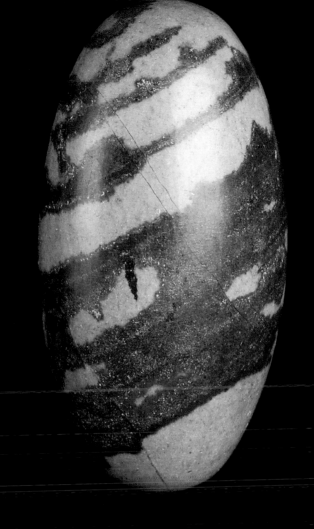

Place a Shiva Lingam over the base
and sacral chakras to stimulate
the integration of masculine and
feminine energy currents and
awaken creative kundalini power.

Shungite

- **Chakra correspondences:** Earth star, base, higher heart (thymus)
- **Physiological correspondences:** Cellular metabolism; neurotransmitters; immune, digestive, and filtration systems; enzyme production; detoxification; antioxidant; antibacterial; anti-inflammatory; antihistamine; pain relief
- **Vibration:** Earthy

LEGENDARY POWER

Shungite's shielding power arises from its unique formation. A rare, noncrystalline carbon mineral, it is composed of hollow fullerenes called "Buckyballs" and contains virtually all the minerals in the periodic table. It may have been instrumental in creating life on this planet. Fullerenes empower nanotechnology, being excellent geothermal and electromagnetic conductors, and yet shield from EMF emissions. Scientists around the world are investigating this mineral's full potential.

This mysterious stone is found in one small area of northern Russia: Karelia. Carbon-based minerals normally arise from decayed organic matter, such as ancient forests, yet Shungite is at least two billion years old, a period before organic life was established. One theory suggests an enormous meteorite hit the Earth and seeded Shungite into the crater in which Lake Onega later formed. Another says microorganisms were already swimming in a soupy sea, and the seabed formed the Shungite deposit. Although the lake is highly polluted, its water is purified by the Shungite bed—and the water has been used in a healing spa for hundreds of years.

HEALING POWER

Shungite-infused water is traditionally drunk two or three times a day to eliminate free radicals and pollutants. According to anecdotal evidence, it acts as an antibacterial and antiviral, preventing or lessening common cold symptoms. The water also heals sore throats, burns, cardiovascular diseases, blood disorders, allergies, asthma, gastric disturbances, diabetes, arthritis and osteoarthritis, kidney and liver disorders, gallblad-der dysfunction, auto-immune diseases, pancreatic disorders, impotence, and chronic fatigue syndrome. Place a Shungite pyramid by the bed to counteract insomnia and headache and eliminate the physiological effects of stress.

TRANSFORMATIONAL POWER

Shungite works at a deep physical level to restore balance to the body—or purity to water. It transforms water into a biologically active substance while simultaneously removing harmful microorganisms and pollutants. Shungite absorbs that which is hazardous to health: pesticides, free radicals, bacteria, viruses, EMF, Wi-Fi, microwaves, and other emissions. It boosts everything that is beneficial for physical well-being, turn-ing water into a life-enhancing essence that powerfully supports the immune system. Shungite also restores emotional equilibrium and transforms stress into a potent ener-getic recharge. (Note: Shungite is a rapid absorber of negative energy and pollutants, so clean it frequently and place it in the sun to recharge. Immerse it in water for at least forty-eight hours to activate the water.)

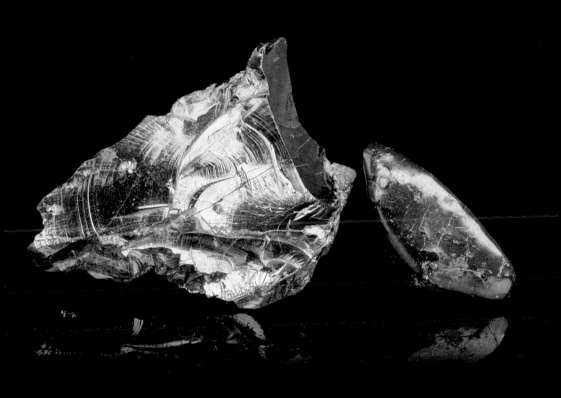

Wear Shungite or place it on the
source of electromagnetic frequency
emissions, such as computers and
cell phones, to eliminate their
detrimental effects.

Smoky Quartz

- **Chakra correspondences:** Earth star, base; cleanses all chakras and shields the aura
- **Physiological correspondences:** Abdomen, legs, feet, muscles, assimilation of minerals, fluid regulation, detoxification, and nervous, reproductive, and elimination systems
- **Vibration:** Earthy and high

LEGENDARY POWER

Sacred to the ancient Druids and Celts, Smoky Quartz symbolized the potent dark power of Earth gods and goddesses. A large Smoky Quartz forms part of the Scepter of Power of the Scottish royal regalia. The stone was an essential ingredient in a magician's tool kit. Dr. Dee, Queen Elizabeth I's seer, had a Smoky Quartz scrying ball for connecting to the lower worlds, controlling the spirits there, and adjusting the course of history. Smoky Quartz shields against psychic attack and transmutes negative energies. Today it is invaluable for absorbing electromagnetic smog, including Wi-Fi emanations and geopathic stress.

Morion is the ancient Scottish name for dark Smoky Quartz, and Pliny speaks of *mormorion*, a transparent deep black crystal. Morions are rare, naturally irradiated, intense black Smoky Quartzes, usually with dolomite or other minerals attached that synergistically enhance its shielding and detoxifying properties. Morions gently heal emotional conditions and overcome lack of trust. Other black Quartzes may have been artificially irradiated and can be radioactive. The "like heals like" principle, however, suggests the energetic resonance of naturally irradiated ones can, if used with care, neutralize toxicity from radiation sources or treatments.

Cairngorm, another Scottish-named stone, is a yellowish Citrine-like Smoky Quartz that brings light into the heart of darkness. My own power ring is a Cairngorm, inherited from my mentor Christine Hartley, a colleague of Dion Fortune, who was active in restoring magical awareness to Britain. I value it highly for its power to help me safely traverse dark places to seek the light and for its ability to synthesize alpha, beta, and theta brainwaves during meditation and journeying.

HEALING POWER

This versatile healing crystal carries the underlying properties of Quartz. It works on the kidneys and other organs of elimination to energetically remove toxins from the body. An excellent grounding stone for rebalancing the body, Smoky Quartz strengthens underlying core stability and prevents healing crises from occurring.

TRANSFORMATIONAL POWER

Smoky Quartz's phenomenal power lies in its ability to transmute negative energies, purifying and returning them as core stability and energetic grounding. It is invaluable in healing layouts or for environmental healing. If your survival instincts are low, if you feel drained of energy or depleted by conditions around you, Smoky Quartz's psychological strength restores your vigor and shines light on the gifts that hide in the shadows of your inner being. (See Brandenberg, Elestial, and Herkimer, pages 60, 84 and 104.)

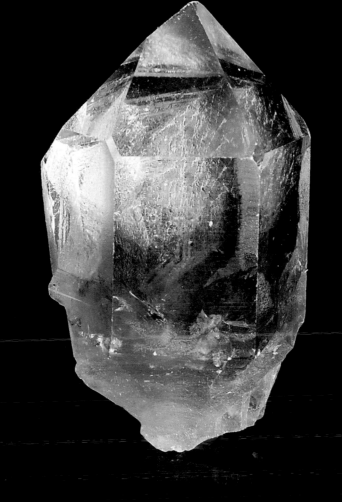

In a healing grid, Smoky Quartz
absorbs disharmonious environmental
energy. With the point facing out, it
transmutes negative energy and with
the point facing in, it draws in
healing light.

Spirit Quartz

- **Chakra correspondences:** Earth, solar plexus, crown, soul star, stellar gateway; cleanses and opens all chakras
- **Physiological correspondences:** Cellular memory, detoxification, skin
- **Vibration:** High

LEGENDARY POWER

A comparatively new find from South Africa, Spirit Quartz is now becoming rare. With tiny points covering an internal core, Spirit Quartz is the perfect metaphor for the holistic, dynamic, holographic consciousness within each of us. The crystal reminds us that the power of the whole is greater than the individuals who comprise it, and that we are all one interconnected spirit.

Facilitating connection to expanded consciousness, this crystal opens the third eye and takes you journeying into other realms. Particularly in its smoky form, it is the perfect accompaniment for a dying person on the journey through death. It encourages awareness of the soul's needs, showing what must be released before the soul can separate from the physical or subtle bodies. Spirit Quartz then comforts the bereaved with the knowledge that spirits are ultimately reunited.

Spirit Quartz carries universal love. It helps you pinpoint important karmic connections and facilitates healing the ancestral line. A Spirit Quartz cluster is particularly helpful for bonding groups who offer spiritual service to the planet.

HEALING POWER

The perfect tool for multidimensional healing, Spirit Quartz focuses high-frequency energy at its point while radiating healing energy in all directions. Acting as a healing wand to pull dis-ease and negative energy out of the body or the aura, it instills light into the resultant spaces. With the assistance of an experienced crystal worker, it seals the aura after soul retrieval has taken place.

Spirit Quartz stimulates the cells to remember their innate perfection and switches on appropriate DNA potential to bring about cellular healing. Placed over the ovaries, it may enhance fertility; over the base chakra, it encourages detoxification. Spirit Quartz-infused water makes a useful elixir for bathing skin eruptions. Place this crystal in bathwater to soothe dry skin.

TRANSFORMATIONAL POWER

"Amethyst" Spirit Quartz opens the higher chakras that are a ladder to multidimensions. "Citrine" connects the earth star to the solar plexus chakra and centers you in your own power. "Citrine" releases dependence on material things, opening you to spiritual abundance. Smoky Spirit Quartz guides the soul in the regions beyond death, but also attunes the base chakra with the third eye, anchoring spiritual insight in the everyday world. Use it to remove karmic debris and cleanse the subconscious mind. Flame and Aqua Aura Spirit Quartz are alchemical gifts for the soul, uplifting it and reminding you of your divine roots.

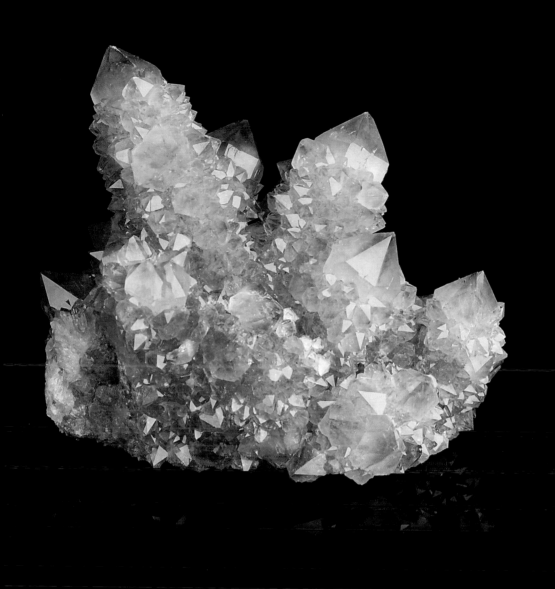

Meditating with Spirit Quartz
reminds you that we are all one
spirit and need to work together
for the good of humanity.

Stibnite

- **Chakra correspondences:** Unites base, sacral, solar plexus, and soma chakras
- **Physiological correspondences:** Stomach, esophagus, eyes, cellular memory, infections, cold sores
- **Vibration:** Earthy, lower worldly, and extraterrestrial

LEGENDARY POWER

Stibnite facilitates separation of the subtle bodies from the physical, so your personal awareness can go traveling. Ancient shamans perceived Stibnite as creating an interface with the multidimensional planes of being. They used it as a portal to pass between the upper and lower worlds where spirits and power animals dwell.

In ancient times, this composite of antimony and sulfur melted at low temperatures, but created a magical, untarnishable, and indissoluble bond for precious metals; it could be combined to create alloys such as pewter. Its most magical power manifested when liberating gold from the base matrix that held it captive.

Stibnite was the basis for kohl, an eye cosmetic that was more than a beauty enhancer. The ancient Greek physician Dioscorides tells us the stone was placed in a lump of dough and baked in the fire until reduced to a cinder. Wine and milk were poured over the cinder to cool it. Pulverized to powder, it was applied to eyes to protect against the fierce sun and prevent ocular diseases. The prophet Mohammed is reputed to have said, "[Stibnite] clears the vision and makes the hair sprout." This stone breaks through illusions, enabling you to see the spiritual reality of All That Is.

HEALING POWER

Although still sometimes used as a medication, Stibnite (antimony) is poisonous and should not be taken internally. Today, it is used to release entity possession, especially by extraterrestrial or shadow energies that deplete well-being. A protective shield against energetic invasion from other worlds, Stibnite forms a one-way portal to block entities that do not belong in our galaxy. In tie-cutting ceremonies, it eliminates the hold past partners may have, teaching you to say no. Stibnite releases cords and old belief patterns that have locked you into the past, dissolving rigidity so you can move forward.

TRANSFORMATIONAL POWER

Hold Stibnite to the soma chakra to attract wolf energy and facilitate journeys with this power animal. The crystal reassures you that you are safe in every moment. It allows you to safely transit the shamanic worlds for soul retrieval and karmic healing, dissolving barriers built up in the past and opening you to trust and love. This stone's transformative power turns your inner dross into spiritual gold. It highlights the soul-learning gifts inherent in all your experiences and activates your shamanic power. (Caution: Stibnite is toxic; handle with care and wash hands thoroughly after use.)

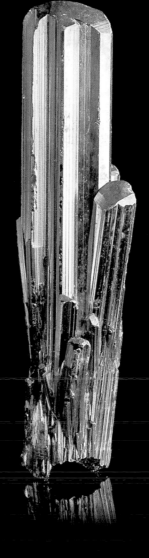

Hold Stibnite to call your power animals and provide a protective energetic shield when journeying out of body, especially when traversing the astral worlds.

Sugilite (Luvulite)

- **Chakra correspondences:** Heart, third eye, crown; aligns all chakras, working from crown to base
- **Physiological correspondences:** Brain, blood, motor function, and nervous and lymphatic systems
- **Vibration:** Earthy and high

LEGENDARY POWER

This powerful stone brings the angels of light and love into the darkest of situations, offering hope and helping you live in truth. Named after the Japanese geologist Ken-ichi Sung, who discovered the stone in Japan in 1944, Sugilite was known in South Africa long before that. Sugilite is one of the great love stones. It infuses the body with light, bringing the ray of spiritual and unconditional love in through the crown chakra and passing it down to the base chakra, aligning as it goes.

Meditating with Sugilite helps answer all the great questions of life: "Why am I here?" "What am I meant to do?" and perhaps most important, "Who am I at my core?" Exploring the foundations of your truth in past and interlives, it helps you recognize and release, with loving forgiveness, causes of dis-ease stemming from the past.

Sugilite is linked to Archangel Michael, the great protector and spiritual warrior.

HEALING POWER

Gentle Sugilite heals shocks and traumas of all kinds. Its manganese base makes it a useful pain reliever, especially for headaches or joints. It may energetically assist psychiatric disorders, neurotransmitter glitches, or brain malfunctions such as dyslexia, dyscalcula, and dyspraxia.

Sugilite relieves emotional turmoil and dis-eases arising from stress or lack of love. Perfect for balancing mind and body, it releases psychosomatic dis-ease. Sugilite is a useful adjunct to the healing process for those suffering from cancer. It lifts despair, calms the emotions, and strengthens trust in the process of recovery. Sugilite helps you understand why you've assumed difficult lessons and recognize the inherent gifts.

TRANSFORMATIONAL POWER

If you have suffered disappointments in the past, Sugilite helps you put these behind you and move on. If you have never fit in or feel too sensitive for your surroundings, this stone helps you realize this is where you belong for the time being.

Sugilite instills love for yourself and awareness that everything is perfect, as is your chosen soul path. A helpful stone for lightworkers who find it difficult to adjust to the vibration of Earth, it connects to the love that the higher self and beings from other dimensions have for the incarnated soul. Sugilite helps you rise above the despair and despondency that negative conditions on Earth can create, so you always hold love and spiritual truth in your heart.

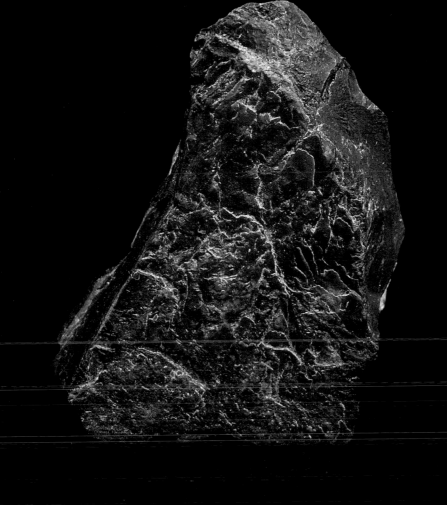

Placed around the head, Sugilite brings the brain hemispheres into balance. It eliminates confusion and realigns the nervous system to create inner peace.

Sunstone

- **Chakra correspondences:** Base, sacral, solar plexus; cleanses and activates all chakras
- **Physiological correspondences:** Immune and autonomous nervous systems, throat, cartilage, muscles, joints
- **Vibration:** Earthy

LEGENDARY POWER

The old lapidaries mention several powerful "stones of the sun," but exact identification is not possible. Today, orangey-red Aventurine and translucent, iridescent, yellow-orange volcanic Feldspar are both known as Sunstone. We are concerned here with the translucent crystal. The ancient Greeks considered Sunstone invigorating. As a magical talisman, it attracted prosperity and good health. Native Americans used Sunstone in medicine wheels to contact the Great Spirit and attract the healing rays of the sun.

Sunstone refracts light, making it possible to locate the sun on a cloudy day. The Vikings are said to have navigated with a Sunstone tied to the ship's mast; this stone was found in ancient Viking graves, suggesting it also guided the soul beyond death to Valhalla. It can act as a spiritual compass for you, too.

Placed over the base and sacral chakras, Sunstone helps you cut ties with previous sexual partners. It removes emotional hooks from the past that may be preventing you from entering into a new relationship.

HEALING POWER

Sunstone traditionally lifts depression and seasonal affective disorder. Keep one in your pocket and handle it frequently. Full of Qi, this regenerative crystal revitalizes the body and the psyche. It heals muscle or joint pain, energetically remobilizing the whole body.

Sunstone is infused with male/yang energy and complements the delicate feminine/yin energy of its sister crystal, Moonstone. The two can be placed at the base chakra—Moonstone on the left and Sunstone on the right—to harmonize the male and female currents as kundalini power rises to the crown.

TRANSFORMATIONAL POWER

Use optimistic Sunstone if you suffer from lack of self-worth or have lost your enthusiasm for life. This crystal does not allow procrastination and gets you back on your path, instilling a deep awareness of your own value. Sunstone is helpful in codependent relationships. If you are prone to being manipulated by others or continually sacrifice yourself to someone else's needs, Sunstone teaches you to say "no" and do only what is appropriate. A stone of self-empowerment, Sunstone lets your true self shine.

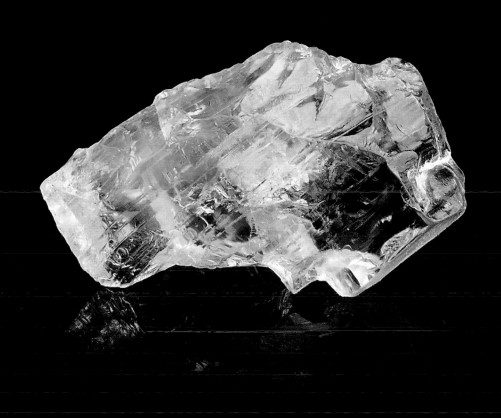

Placed on the solar plexus, Sunstone
removes negative emotional
conditioning and memories, so you
can fulfill your destiny as a joyful
child of the sun.

Tanzanite (Lavender-Blue Zoisite)

- **Chakra correspondences:** Soma; links higher crown to base chakra
- **Physiological correspondences:** Cellular memory, hair, skin, head, throat, chest, spleen, pancreas, kidneys, nervous system
- **Vibration:** High to exceptionally high when genuine

LEGENDARY POWER

Tanzanite is the lavender-blue form of Zoisite. Zoisite was first identified in 1805 by geologist Baron Sigmund Zois von Edelstein in the Saualpe Mountains, Austria. It wasn't until 1967, however, that Manuel D'Souza, while prospecting in Tanzania, was shown what was later named Tanzanite. According to local Masai herders, a lightning strike had set fire to the grass; once the fire was out, they found the crystal scattered around the site. In 1970, Tiffany jeweler Henry Platt named the gem Tanzanite as a marketing ploy. It quickly became a favorite for healing and jewelry, although it is a rare crystal and much of it is artificially created.

In keeping with its origins, Tanzanite is a gem of transmutation; it brings Christ consciousness into the Earth's vibrational field to assist the expansion process. With the stone's assistance, you can read the Akashic Record for your soul, ascertaining your true vocation and the reasons behind the choices you have made on your life path.

Tanzanite may be too strong for sensitive people—it generates a rapid psychic download that can overwhelm the mind. If this occurs, remove it immediately and replace with Smoky Quartz or polished Hematite to realign your energies. When working with Tanzanite again, keep Smoky Quartz at your feet to anchor your soul into your body and ground high-dimensional energies into the Earth. If Tanzanite opens your mind to a telepathic influx, use Healer's Gold or Apatite to create an interface between you and other minds. Place Banded Agate on the third eye if you wish to shut off the telepathy.

HEALING POWER

Tanzanite works best at the nonphysical level to adjust the vibrations of the subtle bodies; from there, it reprograms neural pathways in the brain and cellular memory. This crystal facilitates multidimensional cellular healing that is then reflected in the physical body. It transforms karmic wounds and spiritual dis-ease, lifting depression and raising the body's well-being.

Tanzanite encourages stressed-out people to take time for themselves. It smoothes fluctuations of physical energy. It combines well with Danburite and Iolite for karmic healing.

TRANSFORMATIONAL POWER

Tanzanite is plechroic, meaning it gives you glimpses of the unexpected and opens your mind to spiritual realities beyond consensual reality. This brilliant gem teaches you to live from a compassionate heart and an illumined mind, keeping the balance between the two so you can live expansion and enlightenment on Earth.

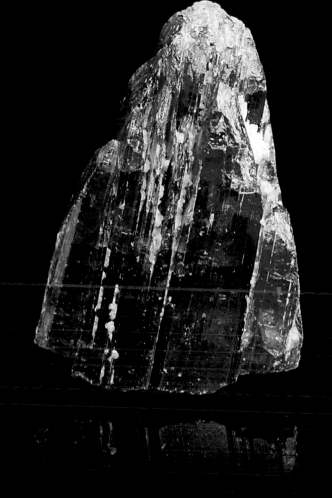

During meditation, Tanzanite connects
your aura to higher dimensions and
the lightbody. It initiates you into
expanded consciousness, facilitates
journeying through multidimensions,
and enhances clairvoyance.

Tiger's Eye

- **Chakra correspondences:** Third eye
- **Physiological correspondences:** Brain, liver, eyes, throat, reproductive organs, bones
- **Vibration:** Earthy and high

LEGENDARY POWER

Roman soldiers wore protective Tiger's Eye amulets to deflect weapons during battle. It appears to have been known as Wolf stone and possibly *oculus belus*, dedicated to the Mesopotamian god Belus, which would make its use ancient indeed. Deemed to be all-seeing, it has long been regarded as a stone of good fortune that protects your resources and defends you against curses.

The bands are created from needles of asbestos fibers or amphibole that have grown synchronously interlayered with quartz. This produces chatoyancy, a rippling, iridescent reflection of light on the surface that looks light when viewed from one direction and dark from another, especially when polished. The chatoyancy or the iron in the stone deflects negative energy.

HEALING POWER

Traditionally, Tiger's Eye heals eye diseases and enhances night vision—it helps you see like a cat in the dark. It rebalances the body on all levels. In Chinese medicine, it restores harmony between yin and yang energies. One stone placed on either side of the head energetically rebalances the brain's hemispheres. Crystal workers use Tiger's Eye to assist digestion, lower blood pressure, and stimulate repair of broken bones. Placed over the reproductive organs, it may encourage fertility and resolve dis-ease arising from past experiences. Placed over the lower chakras, it stimulates the rise of kundalini. As Tiger's Eye holds the energy of the sun, it may aid seasonal affective disorder and depression.

TRANSFORMATIONAL POWER

Tiger's Eye teaches integrity and right use of power. If you have misused, abused, or failed to take hold of your power in the past, this stone shows you how to let power flow through you for the good of all. If you are spaced out and uncommitted or overly proud and willful, wearing it develops your personal will assertively but sensitively. If you find it difficult to remain optimistic, particularly when things seem to be going well, carrying Tiger's Eye helps you trust in the future and set realistic goals for yourself. This stone balances your needs with others' and promotes creative compromise.

Golden Tiger's Eye lets you make decisions from a place of reason rather than emotion. Red Tiger's Eye overcomes lethargy and gets you moving. Blue Tiger's Eye relieves stress. Red stimulates the metabolism, Blue sedates it. Hawk's Eye is traditionally a stone of protection and abundance that facilitates insight and inner vision.

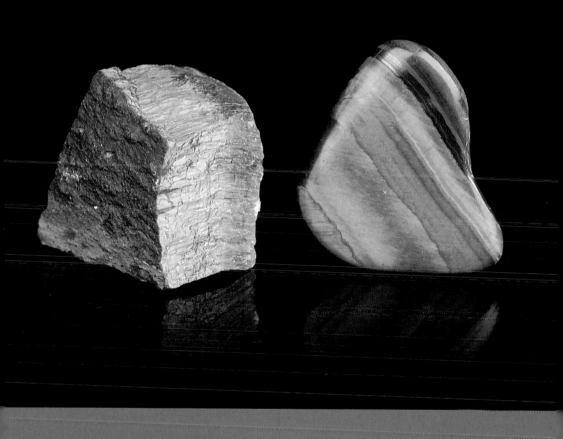

Grid Tiger's Eye or Hawk's Eye
around your home to attract
abundance and health. It also
deflects anything that draws off
or absorbs your abundance.

Topaz

- **Chakra correspondences:** Solar plexus, throat
- **Physiological correspondences:** Eyes, cellular structures, gallbladder; digestive, endocrine, and nervous systems
- **Vibration:** Earthy to high (depends on color)

LEGENDARY POWER

Many legends exist about Topaz, although originally the name also encompassed Peridot and Malachite. Topaz's power comes from its connection to the sun. Its name derives from the Sanskrit word for fire, which suggests its vibrant properties. Some say it was named after Topazios, an island in the Red Sea that was always shrouded in fog. Under the principle of cosmic sympathy and antipathy, this may be connected to Topaz's reputation for clarity—the crystal drives away mental confusion and assists in finding your own inner riches.

Traditionally, Topaz harnessed the power of the sun. Its color was also said to wax and wane with the moon. Pyroelectric, when rubbed vigorously it generates an electrical charge, which may be why it is so efficient at recharging the aura, energizing the physical body, and motivating the psyche.

Topaz symbolizes love, a gentle nature, friendship, and fidelity, and is said to bestow courage and wisdom. A gift of a Topaz amulet kept a beloved safe. According to Agrippa, it had enmity against "spiritual heats," such as lust and other "excesses of love," and guarded against covetousness. It also bestowed power over wild animals.

Topaz is a stone for Archangels Michael and Raziel, keeper of the mysteries. It has dominion over the Archangel realm in one ancient lapidary, over the Cherubim in another. According to the Archbishop of Mainz, it had the power to instill "ardent contemplation of the prophecies."

HEALING POWER

In the tenth century, Topaz was known for its power in healing eye diseases, a quality reiterated by Hildegard of Bingen, who recommended bathing the eyes with Topaz-infused water to overcome dimness of vision. In 1584, Jerome Cardan assured that he had tested the powers of Topaz and it cured insanity—apothecaries sold powdered Topaz as an antidote to madness. Today, it is said to stimulate digestion, assist assimilation of nutrients, and reveal the past-life pattern behind anorexia. Golden Topaz is a useful battery for recharging the body and overcoming nervous exhaustion.

TRANSFORMATIONAL POWER

Topaz brings joy and abundance into your life and attunes you to the true vibrancy of your soul. Natural Blue Topaz helps you live in accordance with your aspirations, rather than following those of other people. It lets you release lifescripts you didn't write so you can live your truth.

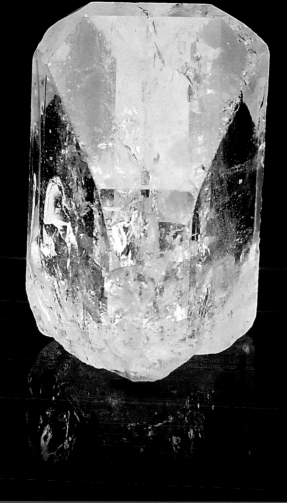

Wear Blue Topaz at your throat
to verbalize your feelings. It
connects to the angels of wisdom
and truth, and takes you into
interdimensional consciousness.

Trigonic Quartz

- **Chakra correspondences:** Higher heart (thymus), soma, soul star, stellar gateway, and higher chakras beyond
- **Physiological correspondences:** Brain, lymphatic system and fluid balance, kidneys, joints, the soul and lightbodies
- **Vibration:** Exceptionally high

LEGENDARY POWER

An initiatory crystal of multidimensional awareness, Trigonic Quartz holds the essence of star beings. Oscillators of energy, Trigonics are psychotronic, forming a supercomputer based on plasma molecules with all crystals communicating no matter where they may be—they function like a hive-mind, spreading across vast distances.

Having made themselves available to assist the evolution of human consciousness, their aim is to eliminate conflict in all its manifestations, personal and collective, inner and outer. The crystals have requested their energy be transferred to water throughout the planet to dissolve the war gene encoded into the human energy system. Trigonics bring conflicts—in yourself or in a group—to the surface for resolution.

The triangles etched into the faces of Trigonics are like cosmic DNA soul encoding. Trigonics create a powerful transformational wave that carries souls, represented by the triangles, through transition to the afterlife or through birth onto Earth. Holding this crystal takes you into multidimensions to view your soul's journey and your purpose.

HEALING POWER

It is essential to release blockages and toxicity from the physical and energy bodies prior to working with Trigonic Quartz or catharsis occurs. The purification process cannot be short-circuited or evaded. Trigonics work mainly on the etheric blueprint, but may also balance the flow of fluid through the body and recalibrate neurotransmitters. Trigonic-infused water made in a Tibetan singing bowl contains potent healing power, purifying and harmonizing the fluid balance in your body. Sound the bowl to transfer the vibration to water, then pour it into a bath, river, or sea.

TRANSFORMATIONAL POWER

Trigonics facilitate movement between levels of reality, expanding your soul to rejoin the holographic oversoul that is consciousness. The crystal creates a calm core around which everything flows—hold it if you feel trapped on Earth. An excellent journeying crystal, Trigonic takes you into a vast interdimensional and interstellar way of being, allowing you to be "here" and "there" simultaneously, knowing all is one. Trigonic keeps you in the moment, reconnected to your higher purpose. By reintegrating soul fragments, it helps you renegotiate soul-group contracts. Once you have experienced the totality of All That Is with this crystal, your vibratory rate is permanently changed to a higher frequency that enables you to midwife others' souls and shifts of consciousness. (Note: Other high-vibration crystals may display etched triangular, Trigonic markings and can be used as stepping-stones to multidimensional reality. *See also cover image.*)

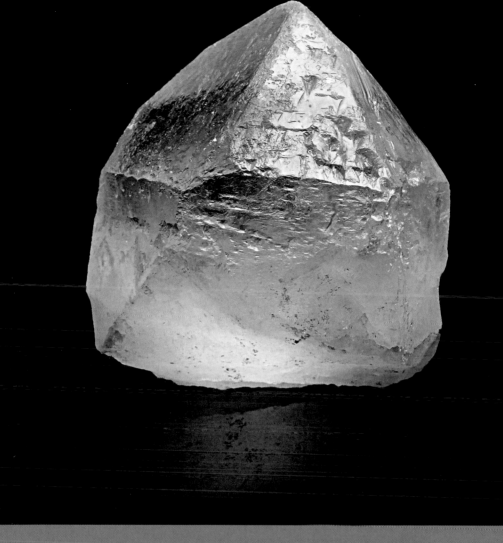

HARNESSING THE POWER

Meditating with Trigonic
facilitates a theta brainwave state
that creates the potential for deep
healing and restructuring of body,
beliefs, and realities.

Tugtupite

- **Chakra correspondences:** Heart, higher heart (thymus), heart seed
- **Physiological correspondences:** Heart and circulation, reproductive system, metabolism, hormone production
- **Vibration:** Exceptionally high

LEGENDARY POWER

A powerful heart healer, Tugtupite reaches the highest of vibrations and brings in unconditional love. It shows you the value of self-love and teaches that Earth is where we learn to master our emotions, staying centered within them rather than repressing, controlling, or being overwhelmed by feelings.

Tugtupite has been known to the Greenland Inuits for millennia. Its name comes from *tuttupit*: reindeer blood. According to Inuit legend, Tutu, a young reindeer herder went into the mountains to give birth. As her sacred blood fell, Tugtupite formed. In sympathetic magic, Tugtupite resonates with the life-giving properties of blood and the potent force blood carries throughout the body. Another Inuit legend says lovers cause the stone to glow fiery red with the heat of their passion—a reference to Tugtupite's tenebrescence: its color intensifies with heat or sunlight. Tugtupite also fluoresces bright red under ultraviolet light. The Inuit say the stone awakens forgotten love and stimulates libido and passionate enthusiasm in everyday life.

Tugtupite literally accesses a new dimension of love, infusing it into the physical world. If you are affected by other people's anger, placing Tugtupite a hand's width under your right armpit protects you. By transmuting the anger into love and forgiveness, Tugtupite sends it back as pink light that gently surrounds the source to bring about a change of attitude. Place Tugtupite over your heart if someone else's strong feelings "mug" you. It cuts off emotional blackmail and people who tug inappropriately on your heartstrings, making you feel emotionally secure. It transforms rage or impotence into powerful creativity, and stimulates your ability to change things for the better. Placed over the heart seed chakra, Tugtupite aligns it with your heart and mind so love is expressed in every moment, in each deed and thought.

HEALING POWER

Tugtupite energetically heals heart, blood, circulation, and blood-rich organs. Perfect for emotional healing, it regulates metabolic and hormonal systems and lifts seasonal affective disorder. Tugtupite's white portion has been noted to turn black in the presence of cancer and toxins.

TRANSFORMATIONAL POWER

Tugtupite teaches you to be emotionally independent yet interdependent, sharing mutual love and support. It says you and you alone are responsible for your happiness or unhappiness. While showing how you create your well-being with the power of your heart and mind, it may generate a gentle emotional catharsis that releases grief so unconditional love expresses itself in your life.

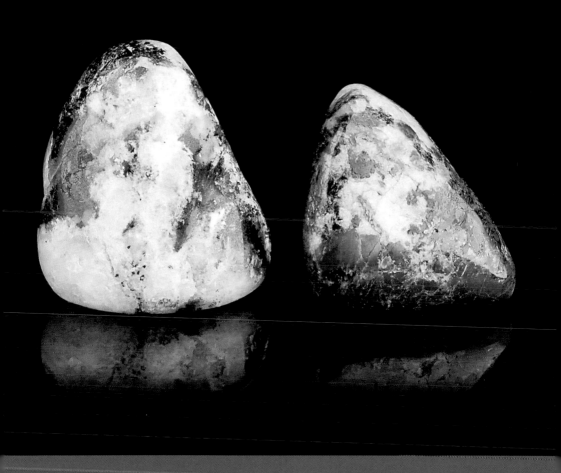

Program Tugtupite to send healing
and peace to the world—especially
areas of ethnic conflict—and to
teach the power of love for all
humanity.

Turquoise

- **Chakra correspondences:** Throat, third eye
- **Physiological correspondences:** Throat, eyes, tissue, cells, immune system, energy meridians, assimilation of nutrients, pain relief
- **Vibration:** High

LEGENDARY POWER

Turquoise was sacred to the Egyptian goddess Hathor (Venus) and imbued with her protective magic. For thousands of years, the desert peoples of the Sinai traded turquoise beads. Sacred also to the Aztecs and native peoples of the Americas, according to Pueblo legend, Turquoise stole its color from the sky and represents humanity's cosmic origins. In the language of gemstones, Turquoise symbolizes cheerfulness of the soul. Universally regarded as a bringer of peace and good luck, it was considered a potent antidote to the evil eye and a fortunate stone for actors and singers.

An Arabic proverb states, "A turquoise given by a loving hand carries with it happiness and good fortune." Hindu tradition says if you set eyes on a Turquoise on the day after seeing the new moon, you will enjoy immeasurable wealth. The powers of abundance and protection feature strongly in legends surrounding this stone. Horses' bridles were set with Turquoise to ensure no accidents befell the riders—the stone was believed to absorb any harm directed toward the wearer.

HEALING POWER

In the Middle Ages, Turquoise was used to heal sore throats and headaches and was said to lose its color in the presence of illness. According to early crystal lore, drinking Turquoise-infused water alleviated urine retention. Today it is said to strengthen the immune system and subtle meridians, regenerate tissue, and encourage assimilation of nutrients. A pain reliever and anti-inflammatory, it may aid cramps, arthritis, and similar dis-eases. Wear Turquoise to alleviate physical or mental exhaustion or to lift depression caused by difficult circumstances.

Turquoise exemplifies the homeopathic principle "like heals like," that is, a substance given in an infinitesimal "energetic signature" dose alleviates a condition it would cause if given in a large dose. It contains phosphoric acid, which in a large dose would sear the throat, but for thousands of years, gentle Turquoise has been prescribed to soothe sore throats. Turquoise also contains traces of iron, noted for its protective qualities, and copper, prized for its anti-inflammatory properties.

TRANSFORMATIONAL POWER

Turquoise lets you explore past lives to find the primary source of a martyred attitude or self-sabotage. If you are pessimistic, it teaches you to focus on solutions rather than problems or the past. This stone dispels negative belief patterns and removes toxic energy, reminding you that you are a spiritual being who happens to be having a human learning experience.

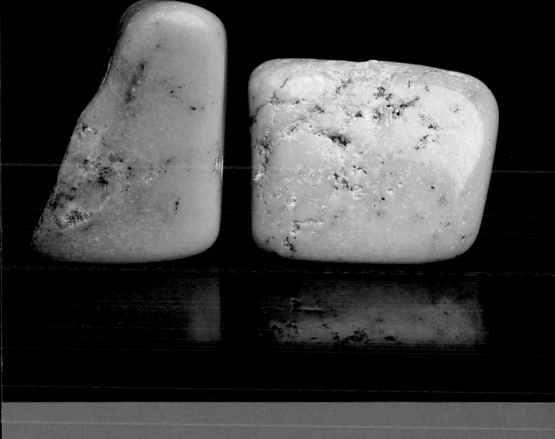

Placed over the throat chakra, Turquoise releases inhibitions and vows from the past that prevent you from fully expressing yourself.

Zincite

- **Chakra correspondences:** Base and sacral, others according to color
- **Physiological correspondences:** Kidneys, skin, hair, prostate gland, heart, fallopian tubes, assimilation, hormonal balance, cellular processes, energy meridians, and immune and electrical systems
- **Vibration:** Medium to high

LEGENDARY POWER

Natural Zincite is rare. Most Zincite is formed by an alchemical sublimate crystallizing inside the fiery chimneys of smelting plants. Even natural Zincite was formed by metamorphosis: a change of structure. A powerful metaphor for physical and spiritual transmutation, Zincite is a potent healing tool valued for its range of colors and energetic frequencies.

Zincite is beneficial if you are a kinesthetic (body-feeling) person who wants to be more in tune with your gut instincts. A great deal of intuition shows itself through bodily signals; wearing Zincite alerts you to these and helps you interpret them correctly.

Use this crystal to remove hypnotic commands instilled by other people and to disconnect undue mental influences that unconsciously control your behavior. It draws together like-minded people as a support group. Red Zincite is particularly helpful for boosting the manifestation process—program it to bring you abundance and prosperity. All Zincite acts as a first aid remedy for shock or trauma.

HEALING POWER

As suggested by the name, Zincite contains zinc, essential for cellular metabolism, teeth, bones, skin, and hair. Zinc is necessary for prostate functioning, and Zincite energetically assists the body in metabolizing and assimilating nutrients, supporting the prostate as well as muscles and joints. Red Zincite strengthens energy meridians and the immune system, overcoming energetic depletion. It also eases depression and seasonal affective disorder. Yellow Zincite energetically heals bladder and kidney infections. Because the crystal may rebalance the hormonal system, it is useful for menopause and PMS. It is worth experimenting with the different colors to assess which stone is most appropriate at any particular time, as hormone levels can fluctuate.

Zincite's healing power works according to its color: Red energizes, restructures, and stabilizes; Yellow and Green rebalances and calms. Zincite anchors the subtle and lightbodies into the physical body. It also draws out toxic energy or underlying thought patterns that can create dis-ease.

Meditating with Zincite can reveal the causes of phobias and assist in reprogramming your mind. It is an excellent stone for tapping the meridians in energy-based techniques such as EFT and NLP as it anchors the changing energy into the physical body.

TRANSFORMATIONAL POWER

A potent transmutor of energy, Zincite detoxifies and synthesizes body, psyche, and soul. By reminding your soul of its purpose in incarnating, it helps you find your inner strength and manifest your creativity.

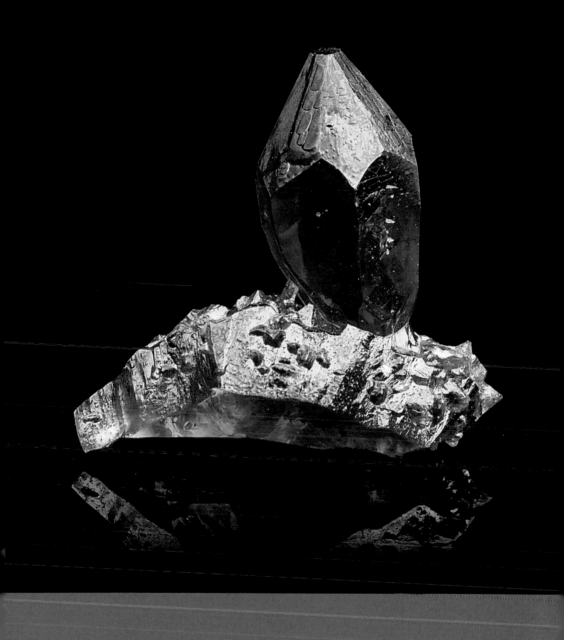

Placed over the base or sacral chakra, Zincite synthesizes personal power and creativity, empowering regeneration and manifestation on every level.

Alchemical marriage: a blending of inner energy that merges masculine and feminine currents into androgynous unity and infuses a higher level of Qi (life force) into the body and spiritual awareness.

All That Is: spirit, source, the divine, the sum total of everything, quantum consciousness.

Alfonso Lapidary (The Lapidary of King Alfonso X The Learned): a twelfth-century Spanish book of stones that preserved ancient Greek and Arabic crystal and astrological lore.

Ancestral line patterns: beliefs, behaviors, and attitudes passed through the family from earlier generations. Within the physical body, cells contain molecular gates that can be blocked by ancestral genetic memory. If the memory is removed, DNA potential is activated.

Ascension: see Expansion process

Cellular memory: beliefs, attitudes, traumas, and patterns ingrained within the cells that create present-day reality.

Central channel: an energetic tube running up the center of the body (close to the spine) linking the chakras and expanded consciousness. The pathway for kundalini power. Energetic pathways branch off the central channel to take subtle energy to every part of the physical body.

Chakra: an energy vortex or linkage point between the physical and subtle bodies and multidimensional consciousness.

Correspondence: an ancient system of affiliations and reflections based on the principle of "as above, so below." It is not that what happens above affects below, rather that what is below is a reflection of what is above and vice versa: There is an energetic two-way resonance or "energetic signature."

Cosmic consciousness: connection to All That Is.

Crystal-infused water: see Essence

Dantien: a small, spirally rotating sphere that sits on top of the sacral chakra. It is a major powerhouse and power-store for the body, acting as a higher resonance of the creativity of the sacral chakra.

Dis-ease: a subtle disharmony resulting from energetic disturbance, mental constructs, emotional blockages, karma, or physiological imbalance that, if not corrected, leads to physical or mental illness.

Drusy: a coating of tiny crystals over the main body of a larger crystal, usually but not necessarily of the same type.

Earth healing: rectifying energy distortion in the Earth's energy field with the use of stones, often laid in a grid pattern.

Electromagnetic smog/EMF: a subtle but detectable field from computers and other electronic devices, power lines, and power stations that can have a detrimental effect on sensitive people.

Energy download: an influx of energy from the higher vibrations/dimensions of consciousness.

Energy signature: every living being (including crystals) has a unique vibratory force field that is its energy signature; some are high and fast, others lower and slow.

Entity attachment/removal: discarnate beings attached to and feeding off the aura of a living person. Entities may be human or extraterrestrial and can be removed by skilled crystal workers with the assistance of suitable crystals.

Essence/crystal infused-water: the energetic vibrations of a crystal can be transferred to water by immersing a crystal in spring water and placing in sunlight. The essence is rubbed on the skin or placed in bathwater. An essence can be bottled with two-thirds brandy or vodka as a preservative.

Etheric body/energy body/aura: the subtle vibrational biomagnetic sheath that surrounds the physical body and accesses multilevels of awareness.

Etheric blueprint: the energetic pattern from which the physical body is created. Karmic wounds, attitudinal karma, mental constructs, ancestral inheritance, and energetic disruptions in the blueprint create dis-ease, which ultimately manifests in the physical body.

Expansion process: extension, expansion, and evolution of consciousness through an increase in self-mastery and self-awareness that raises the spiritual and material vibrations of the physical body, so that it grounds and integrates multi-dimensional consciousness within it. The expansion process does not entail ascending bodily off the planet; it brings expanded consciousness to earth via the lightbody through alignment of mind, body, and spirit.

Geopathic stress: toxic stress created in the Earth by underground water, power lines, or negative energy flow.

Grid: to lay out stones in a specific pattern to bring about balance or protection. The physical and subtle bodies and the Earth have natural meridian energy grids that maintain well-being. Dis-ease occurs when these are disrupted, blocked, or out of balance.

Grounding: making a strong connection between the soul, subtle energy bodies, the physical body, and the Earth; or anchoring energies in the Earth.

High vibration: high-vibration crystals resonate at a lighter, finer, higher frequency that reaches multidimensional and interdimensional consciousness.

Ill-wishing/psychic attack: jealous or envious thoughts or concentrated, malevolent intention to do someone harm.

Implants: energetic "hooks" or mental imperatives planted in the energy body by an outside source.

Infused water: see Essence

Inner dimensions/levels/being: core awareness that encompasses intuition, metaphysical abilities, feelings, emotions, the subconscious mind, and subtle energetic processes and "spaces."

Journeying: traveling in the subtle bodies to other dimensions or worlds, leaving the physical body behind.

Karma/karmic: a continuous, dynamic process of causation and balance brought about by previous experience and the karmic seeds from past lives. Karma is created in every moment. Karmic enmeshment means entanglements that continuously repeat.

Kundalini: the energy of creation. A subtle electromagnetic sexual and spiritual force that resides in the base of the spine which, when activated, rises up through the central channel to reach cosmic consciousness. It creates orgasmic ecstasy in every cell of the body, infusing it with enlightenment.

Kythe: a two-way process of exchanging information with beings in higher dimensions.

Lightbody: a subtle energetic and spiritual body that resonates at a high frequency and which forms a vehicle for higher, multidimensional consciousness and spirit.

Like heals like: this ancient homeopathic principle says a substance that would cause a condition if taken in a large dose alleviates the problem when given in an infinitesimal "energetic signature" dose.

Meridian: subtle energy channel within the physical or subtle bodies or in the Earth.

Multidimensional/interdimensional realities/dimensions/consciousness: lighter, finer, higher frequencies that encompass galactic, cosmic, and other levels of consciousness.

Physiological: the physical construction of and the biochemical, chemical, and electrical processes operating within cells and organs of the physical body.

Pliny: Roman geographer who wrote about the properties of stones, giving insight as to how they were used in ancient times.

Portal: an energetic gateway between dimensions that are vibrating at different rates. A portal links nonphysical hyperspace and the matrix of the material world and infuses it with quantum consciousness.

Psychic vampirism: pulling on someone else's energy to feed one's own.

Quantum consciousness: awareness of multidimensional and interdimensional functions and processes of the cosmos and consciousness itself.

Reframing: seeing a past event in a more positive, life-enhancing way that can change present and future outcomes.

Shadow qualities/energies: qualities and experiences that have been repressed and pushed out of conscious awareness.

Shamanic anchor: a grounding cord going from the base and earth star chakras deep into the Earth to gently hold the soul in incarnation and enable safe return after journeying.

Soul contracts: agreements made between souls in previous lives or the space between lives—the interlife.

Soul fragmentation: pieces of soul energy that have remained fixed in past-life trauma, joy, or in the post-death state.

Soul group: a group of soul beings with a complementary vibratory field who have traveled together throughout time and beyond.

Star beings: energy forms from elsewhere in the galaxy that resonate with a particular star or galactic location and a specific crystal.

Theophrastus: ancient Greek philosopher and naturalist who wrote the earliest extant scientific treatise on stones and their properties in the fourth century B.C.E.

Twelve-strand DNA: crystal lore suggests humanity originally had twelve strands to the DNA, giving greater potential for linking to other dimensions.

Vibrational shift: a change from a lower to higher energy frequency and higher level of consciousness.

FURTHER READING

Judy Hall, *The Crystal Bible Volumes 1 and 2* (London: Godsfield Press/Walking Stick Press, 2003 and 2009)

Judy Hall, *The Encyclopedia of Crystals* (London: Godsfield Press, and Beverly, Massachusetts: Fair Winds Press, 2007)

Judy Hall, *The Crystal Zodiac: Use Birthstones to Enhance Your Life* (London: Godsfield Press, 2005)

Judy Hall, *The Crystal Experience: Your Complete Crystal Workshop in a Book* (London: Godsfield Press, 2010)

Judy Hall, *Crystal Prosperity* (Lewes: Leaping Hare Press, 2010)

Judy Hall, *Crystal Prescriptions* (Alresford: O Books, 2005)

Judy Hall, *The Astrology Bible* (London: Godsfield Press, 2005)

Judy Hall, *Good Vibrations: Psychic Protection, Energy Enhancement, Space Clearing* (Bournemouth: Flying Horse Publications, 2009)

Judy Hall, *The Soulmate Myth: A Dream Come True or Your Worst Nightmare?* (Bournemouth: Flying Horse Publications, 2010)

Judy Hall, *The Book of Why: Understanding Your Soul's Journey* (Bournemouth: Flying Horse Publications, 2010)

Judy Hall is a successful Mind Body Spirit author with forty-two books to her credit including the million-selling *Crystal Bible (volumes 1 and 2)*. She has been a past-life therapist and karmic astrologer for more than forty years. An internationally known author, psychic, healer, broadcaster, and workshop leader, her books have been translated into fifteen languages. She recently appeared on the *Watkins Review* list of the one hundred most spiritually influential authors.

A trained healer and counselor, Judy has been psychic all her life and has a wide experience of many systems of divination and natural healing methods. Judy has a bachelor of education degree in religious studies with an extensive knowledge of world religions and mythology and a master of arts in cultural astronomy and astrology at Bath Spa University. Her mentor was Christine Hartley (Dion Fortune's metaphysical colleague and literary agent). She runs crystal, past life, and creative writing courses at her home in Dorset.

Her specialities are past-life readings and regression, soul healing, reincarnation, astrology and psychology, divination, and crystal lore. Judy has conducted workshops around the world and has made fifteen visits to Egypt, the subject of her novel *Torn Clouds*. See www.judyhall.co.uk.

Judy Hall would like to thank Robert Simmons of Heaven and Earth for permission to use the trademarked names designated ™ within the text. John Van Rees Sr. and John Van Rees Jr. of Exquisite Crystals are to be congratulated for the wonderful crystal photography and have my gratitude for the introduction to Trigonics and many more marvelous crystals. I also bless David Eastoe of www.petaltone.co.uk, without whose cleansing, recharging, and ally essences I could not continue my crystal work. The translation of Theophrastus's work used throughout this book is by Earle R. Caley and John C. Richards, published by Columbia University, 1956. Their impeccable scholarship is to be applauded as it clarified nomenclature conundrums and highlighted false claims made by later "authorities." The Pliny translation is by D. E. Eichholz, Loeb Classical Library, and *The Lapidary of King Alfonso X The Learned*, by Ingrid Bahler and Katherine Gyekenyesi Gatto. *The Lithica* is taken from the 1864 (first) edition of Charles William King *The Natural History, Ancient and Modern, of Precious Stones and Gems, and of Precious Metals* (it was omitted from later editions). Over the past forty years plus, I have read several hundred books and articles, ancient and modern, about stones, their properties, history, and legends and cannot possibly acknowledge—or even remember—them all, but I thank everyone, especially my workshop participants, for their contribution to my knowledge. Heartfelt thanks also to Skye Alexander for her sensitive editing and thought-provoking questions that made shaping this book a pleasure.

Exquisitecrystals.com began in 1999 as a work of love by John Van Rees Sr. He was joined in the business by his son, John Van Rees Jr., in 2007. John Jr. has held an interest in photography since a very early age, even wining prizes for his photos as young as age 7. All photos attributed to Exquisitecrystals.com in this book were taken by John Van Rees Jr.

John Sr. and Judy Hall have been friends for many years, beginning when she found Exquisitecrystals.com on the web and admired not only the quality specimens but the exceptional photographs. Ms. Hall personally asked for John Van Rees Jr. to photograph the pictures for this book.

Exquisitecrystals.com is located in Vancouver, Washington, USA. You can see their website at www.exquisitecrystals.com.